Made for Paradise

Made for Paradise

God's Original Plan for Healthy Eating, Physical Activity, and Rest

Patricia Hart Terry, PhD, RD, LD

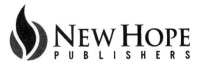

NEW HOPE
PUBLISHERS

Birmingham, Alabama

New Hope® Publishers
P. O. Box 12065
Birmingham, AL 35202-2065
www.newhopepublishers.com

Please be aware that information in this book is provided to supplement the care provided by your physician. It is neither intended nor implied to be a substitute for professional medical advice. Always seek the advice of your physician or other qualified health provider before starting any new health regimen or activity and with any questions you may have regarding a medical condition. The resources included herein are provided for your information and may or may not reflect the opinion of New Hope Publishers.

Library of Congress Cataloging-in-Publication Data

Terry, Patricia Hart, 1949-
  Made for paradise : God's original plan for healthy eating, physical
activity, and rest / Patricia Hart Terry.
     p. cm.
  ISBN-13: 978-1-59669-085-1 (sc)
  1. Health—Religious aspects—Christianity. 2. Nutrition—Religious
aspects—Christianity. 3. Exercise—Religious aspects—Christianity.
4. Rest—Religious aspects—Christianity. 5. Health. 6. Nutrition. 7.
Exercise. 8. Rest. I. Title.
BT732.T47 2007
261.8'321—dc22
                            2006023968

All Scripture quotations, unless otherwise indicated, are taken from the HOLY BIBLE, NEW INTERNATIONAL VERSION®. NIV®. Copyright ©1973, 1978, 1984 by International Bible Society. Used by permission of Zondervan. All rights reserved.

Scripture quotations marked (KJV) are taken from The Holy Bible, King James Version.

ISBN-10: 1-59669-085-2
ISBN-13: 978-1-59669-085-1

N064141 • 0107 • 5M1

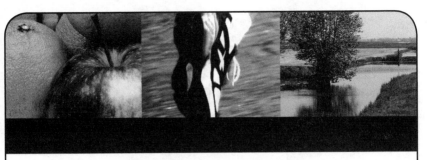

DEDICATION

To my children and grandchildren,

*May we leave you in a world as wonderful as
God intended it to be.*

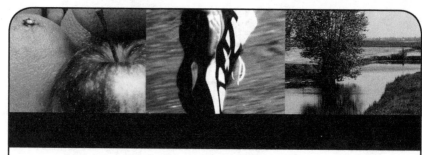

TABLE OF CONTENTS

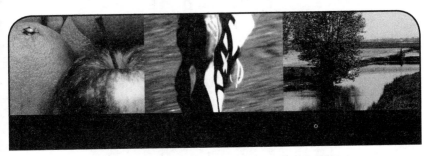

INTRODUCTION

"So why should I read another book about healthy anything? I'm tired of hearing about it. I have information overload as it is. Nothing ever works for me."

Am I reading your mind? I thought so. You are not alone. We hear it on the radio, on TV, from friends, from family, from our doctor; we see it on the Internet, in newspapers, in magazines, in millions of self-help books, and we still don't understand it.

That's the reason I wrote **one more book** about health and wellness. Because when you come down to it, if you have every other resource in the world and don't have health, what do you have? The good news is that you don't have to have a PhD in nutrition, exercise science, and psychology to be healthy. You just have to use common sense—something we seem to have forgotten as a nation.

How do I know this? I know this from gaining 20 extra pounds myself after age 50 and having my blood pressure and blood cholesterol go up with the pounds. After living 11 years in a Third World country as a missionary, purchasing and cooking whole local foods and walking a lot every day of those 11 years, I came back to the processed- and fast-food mecca of the world, America—and drove every mile of every day. The extra pounds didn't take long to creep up, and after menopause, those pounds located in places they had not settled before.

WE HAVE THE ANSWER

Over the last 17 years, I have come to the slow realization that as a Christian, I have had the answer all along, but didn't recognize it. It was so simple I almost missed it. God did not put us here without a guidebook. As I read my Bible to see what God Himself had said about health and wellness, I began to see that He had provided all we need to know about it, because that was His original intention. We can see what God intended in the way He created the world, and in the story of the Garden of Eden. When He made us, He had already made a world for us to live in that would regulate our metabolism by the sun and provide just the right foods for our bodies to function as they should. He gave us physical work to do. He provided a day of rest. That's all we need to know. When I started living by these principles, I lost the weight, I rebuilt muscle, my cholesterol and blood pressure went back down, and I was in the best shape of my life—after 50!

That's why I ask you to go back to Creation's garden with me, back to the paradise of common sense about eating, physical activity, and rest. And since I have invited you along, I'd better introduce myself.

MY CALL

Wife, mother, stepmother, grandmother, daughter, dietitian, missionary, professor, hiker, traveler, cook, reader, student—that describes me in a nutshell! Pat Hart Terry—wife of Bob; mother of Jennifer and Taylor; stepmother of Jean and Brent; grandmother of Karl, Jamey, Kassidi, Jessica, and Drayton; daughter of Jimmy and Gloria. You would think that combination a full-time job in itself, but it's just the beginning!

I was born in Alabama, but my journey has taken me far from my place of birth. I have now come full circle—back to Alabama as a professor of nutrition and dietetics at Samford University. Growing up in a small town near Birmingham didn't stop me from dreaming of being a missionary in a faraway country. Some of my earliest memories are of listening to missionaries on stateside assignment and thinking that would be the most wonderful thing a person could do! After becoming a Christian at an early age, I had my ups and downs learning what it meant to grow in Christ, and I had a turbulent college experience, during which I questioned what I really believed—but "the missionary call" never left. As a junior in college, I finally had the chance to work as a summer missionary in Iowa, and then the next summer, in Israel. Both of these experiences confirmed that call, but the summer of 1972 in Israel sealed the deal!

My junior year in college, I had changed my major from predentistry to nutrition and dietetics. I had been studying nutrition for two years when I spent those four months in Israel. I still recall the Arab names; I still see the faces of the street vendors in the old city; I still smell the roasting pine nuts. All those things were seared into my memory as I realized that the nutritional diseases that I had been studying for two years were right there in front of me, jumping right off the pages of my textbooks into real life! Vitamin A deficiency, scurvy, rickets, protein calorie malnutrition—I saw them in people every day. In those four months, not only did I see the spiritual needs rampant in those faraway places I had dreamed about, but I saw physical needs as well. And so I came home, graduated from college, spent a year in a dietetic internship to become a registered dietitian, got married, went to seminary, went to language school, and then went to Venezuela as a Southern Baptist missionary and worked there as a nutritionist for 11 years.

To tell you the truth, I wanted to go as a missionary to just about anywhere...except Latin America. My two semesters of Spanish in college nearly gave me a nervous breakdown (literally). Having stayed up too late studying for a Spanish final, I collapsed in sobs to the horror of my instructor, who promptly sent me to the infirmary! But God does have a sense of humor, so He sent me back to try again—this time in Costa Rica—for a whole year! Full-time language study was *much* better, but I must confess that I polished off what Spanish I learned in

Costa Rica by watching Venezuelan *novelas* (soap operas). Just my second year in Venezuela, I was asked to teach nutrition classes to the wives of students at the seminary. We struggled through that together, but by the end of the course, I had more of the nutrition vocabulary down and started working with women's groups in the churches. Armed with materials from the Venezuelan Institute of Nutrition and accompanied by a Venezuelan nutritionist much of the time, we began our nutrition education classes for pregnant women and mothers. Of course, my work as a nutritionist went alongside work in the local churches. After my two children were born there, I was able to model the benefits of breast-feeding and proper weaning foods as I went from pillar to post with my children in tow, including traveling to teach nutrition education for missionaries and churches in other Latin American countries. My children marvel at all the countries they have been to with no recollection at all—they were too little to remember.

LIFE IN VENEZUELA

I loved living in Venezuela. I came to love the country. I came to love the people. I learned to love the Latin way of life and mind-set—so different from those in North America. There, relationships and family come first. There, time is relative. Time is taken to spend with children, parents, and siblings. Family is very important. Friends are very important. Time is still taken to *live* every day as you walk (and I emphasize *walk*) from the baker to the meat market to the vegetable and fruit markets. It was in Costa Rica and Venezuela where I first experienced "slow food"—where time was taken to purchase local ingredients from friends, cook the meal with family and friends, and linger at the table and savor the food and the experience. Life in Latin America and many other Third World countries still allows time for healthy eating, physical activity, and rest. Although the Americanized lifestyle in many large Third World cities has changed this, the majority of people in those regions still take time to **live**.

BACK HOME, BUT STILL LIVING THE CALL

I have now been back in Alabama longer than I lived overseas. That is hard to believe. It is also hard to believe that my children are grown, and I now have five grandchildren of my own. What is easy to believe is that my call has not changed—just my location. For 17 years, I have seen the Lord bring Latin America to me in Birmingham. I have continued to go overseas to work in health clinics and on other projects, but through my local church and community service with my students at Samford, my opportunities to minister to the Hispanic population around me—here in America—just continually increase. God is so good!

I do still hike and travel and cook and read and study in my spare time. I also have to intentionally walk extra steps, climb stairs, use my total workout equipment, or do strength training five to six days a week just to fight what midlife tries to do to my body!

At Samford, I teach all levels of classes, from freshman to senior. Throughout the curriculum, I try to emphasize the importance of food in nutrition and dietetics. That may seem strange, but there was a time when even the clinical dietitian forgot that it is all about food. As a profession, we have learned by experience that no matter what a person *should eat* for good health, if it doesn't taste good or is not attractive, *it won't be eaten*—and that's the whole point! We have to actually eat healthy foods to get all the nutritional benefits from them. The science of nutrition forgot about the art of food preparation. Today, it isn't uncommon to find gourmet chefs in the kitchens of many hospitals.

Food—God's bountiful blessing to us—is to be celebrated! For my students at Samford, in seminars, at lectures, and wherever I go, I try to emphasize the importance and relationship of healthy eating, physical activity, and rest to wellness, because they are all interrelated.

THE RETURN TO HEALTHY LIVING—IT'S CATCHING ON!

In the last 17 years, not only have I seen my profession change, I have seen Birmingham and Alabama change, too. Little by little, the importance of locally grown sustainable agriculture is catching on—in Alabama! You can actually find artisan cheeses, yogurt, and ice cream. We have locally grown, grass-fed, organic meat, poultry, eggs, and milk. Local produce is advertised on billboards—**Buy Fresh, Buy Local**—saying it out loud is music to my ears. I long to see the day when I will again know my butcher and baker and farmer by name. Extended-care facilities are encouraging their residents to plant and tend vegetable and flower gardens. Sidewalks have begun appearing in my community, so children can walk to school and residents can walk to shopping centers. Church activity centers now have exercise and strength training for seniors. Internet sites and DVDs galore walk you through aerobic activity and strength training at home.

There is much to celebrate in the progress made. Much more is yet to be done in order to ensure that Americans use common sense again when it comes to healthy living. It wasn't that long ago that our grandparents and great-grandparents knew exactly where their food came from. Life wasn't easy for them, but for the most part, they ate well, even if simply. They worked hard, because they had to. They rested on Sunday, because there was nothing else to do!

As I have studied nutrition and life for 31 years—through earning a bachelor's degree, a master's, and a doctorate and beyond—I have become more and more convinced, as have other researchers, that we really *are* what we eat and do and think. That is why I am passionate about returning to the healthy living and wellness that God intended for His perfect creation. Join me as we look at how we were *made for paradise* and what we all can do to return together!

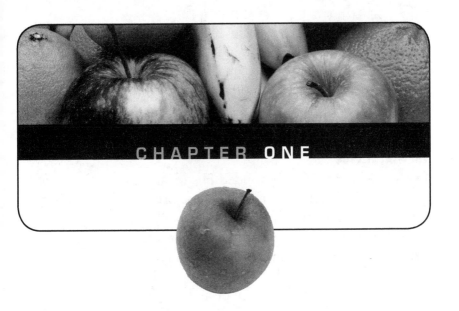

IN THE BEGINNING

As it was in the beginning,
is now, and ever shall be.
—Anonymous, "Gloria Patri"

GOLDEN melons bursting with juice; vine-ripened tomatoes in a rainbow of colors; the sweet perfume of ruby red strawberries; corn, okra, and green beans picked just today, fresh and crisp—where am I? Walking through the local farmers market in July, I'm looking for a place to sit in the shade while I eat my perfect peach. (Yes, I washed it!) I let the juice drip down my chin, onto my fingers, and down to the ground!

There's nothing better on a hot summer's day. I take the time to enjoy each incredible, drippy bite, savoring all the flavor. One might say, "That sounds just like paradise," and I agree.

THE WAY IT WAS

In the beginning, God provided His creation with the basic principles for healthy living, and those principles are **healthy eating, physical activity,** and **rest.** After God made the animals, He made Adam and Eve. He didn't just speak them into being as He did the animals; He made Adam and Eve with His own hands and put them in a beautiful and fruitful garden that He had prepared for them (Genesis 1:27–29 and 2:7–9). His plan was for them to work it and to care for all the plants and trees in the garden (Genesis 2:15), which grew so abundantly. He made their bodies specifically to be able to use energy and nutrients from those foods for physical activity. Best of all, in His perfect world, He walked in the garden with Adam and Eve in joy and restful fellowship and gave us His example of rest (Genesis 2:2–3 and 3:8).

In the beginning, it was heaven on earth—and the perfect balance of healthy eating, physical activity, and rest. God created us to be healthy and well. He made provisions for that in the Creation's garden. After the Fall, however, mankind went its own way. I hate it when we do that! Sin forever changed our world and our relationship with God, who created us for wholeness.

Health fads will come and go. But the original instruction book for our bodies was written in the mind of God before the world began and then literally into our very DNA. God's handprints are all over us. He made our metabolism, hormones, brain chemicals, and muscles—every bodily system—to work with the gifts of nature, food, activity, and rest, which He ordained from the beginning.

The whole **foods** of nature's bounty,
taken in moderation for energy and nutrition,
sustain body systems.

+

Physical **activity** burns the energy and
regulates body systems.

+

Adequate **rest** from
prayer, meditation, relaxation, and sleep
restores and renews body systems.

Food for sustenance, activity for regulation, and **rest for restoration** are good gifts from God, given to us in the beginning to work with our body's design. The abuse of any of these gifts threatens our physical, emotional, and spiritual health.

Your own body has the answers for the wholeness that God intended. Listen to it! Forget the fads, and listen to your Creator and Heavenly Father. By returning to the biblical principles of healthy eating, physical activity, and rest found in Genesis chapters 1 through 3, we can reclaim the lifestyle that God meant for our good. In the New Testament, Paul reminds the Roman and Corinthian believers that our bodies are not our own, they are, in fact, the temple of the Holy Spirit (Romans 8:11; 1 Corinthians 6:19).

THE WAY IT IS

So what's the big deal, you ask? You must be kidding! Just look around. Americans are among the most obese people in the world—yes, in the world. That's the problem we see. The hidden problem is the prevalence of disordered eating, of which obesity is just one extreme. Add to this the heart disease, stroke, cancer, diabetes, and other conditions related to obesity and stress, and you have a lot of unhealthy people on a lot of medication. What's wrong with this picture?

It's just the American way—ask any Texan! The bigger the better; the more the merrier! Americans don't do anything

ay. After all, this is the land of Superman, superstores, and
sizes! The sizes of food portions in restaurants and at home
: increased steadily over the past 30 years, as have the sizes
verage plates and glasses. Since the 1970s, Americans have
n eating more (calories in) and moving less (calories out).
the fast-food revolution took over our country, so did the
uch potatoes, thanks to the technology of TV, computers, and
omputer games.

This is a no-brainer. More energy in plus less energy out is
a math problem a first-grader could solve. We have made a lot
of excuses as a nation; we have tried low-fat, low-carb, and
high-protein diets, plus every diet pill imaginable; but the bottom
line has remained the same. We get heavier and heavier. Add to
that equation the stress factors of American life (a hurried life),
and you have a nation of people in whom heart attacks, high
blood pressure, stroke, diabetes, and renal failure are just waiting to happen. And these diseases are happening at younger and
younger ages and at staggering rates.

In the past 20 years, rates for obesity and type 2 diabetes have
doubled in the American population. In children and adolescents,
these rates have tripled. Alarm bells have finally gone off in almost
every corner of the United States concerning the reality of obese
America and its medical and financial consequences for generations to come. However, because of the spread of sugar and trans
fat–laden processed food around the world and ever-increasing
urbanization, obesity is a growing problem worldwide. Now, overweight people in the world outnumber the malnourished and
hungry people! The World Health Organization (WHO) calls
obesity a global epidemic.

A recent study in France by Kaiser Permanente gives us some
news that would cause even the most casual of gourmands to
shudder! In France, a country with gastronomy and good food
at the heart of its national identity, fast food and the lifestyle
that comes with it are taking over. This fast-food culture that
is quickly changing traditional patterns of eating is also changing the country's health status. For France, which has had the

lowest rate of obesity among nine northern European countries and one of the lowest among westernized countries in the world, these results raise some important social and cultural questions. The French paradox—the French lifestyle that protects against obesity, heart disease, and diabetes—is disappearing. As more and more of the French adopt an American lifestyle that includes fast foods, processed foods, soft drinks, and little or no exercise, a rise in incidence of obesity and diabetes (as began in America nearly 20 years ago) is occurring among that population.

Italy, Greece, Spain, and other previously healthy countries are slowly moving in the same direction. In China, Japan, the Middle East, and Europe, obesity has tripled, especially in cities. Children are leading the way in obesity as they shun traditional healthy foods for fast/processed food and sugary drinks. In addition to eating unhealthy foods, these populations are more sedentary than ever before. TV and video games are also limiting traditional physical activity.

Even the concept of rest is changing in many places in the world. Due to global competition, many banks and offices that used to close for the long lunch hour now stay open. The traditional long lunch and snooze, known as *la siesta*, was once regarded as part of the cultural heritage of Spain and Central and Latin America. Today, however, it is fast becoming an endangered pleasure. Today only a quarter of the population in Spain, mostly those in the hotter southern parts of the country as opposed to the cooler northern regions, are regular siesta takers; the others no longer have time for rest! In addition, more women are working, so those traditionally responsible for cooking the family's full lunch, which is central to that ritual, are too busy to cook and are also eating on the go. Many people in Central and Latin America have adopted similar hurried schedules. The Mexican government recently passed a law limiting lunchtime to one hour, rather than allowing those two- or three-hour lunch breaks, with return to work late in the evening. *¡Qué lástima!* (What a pity!) I lived in Costa Rica and Venezuela long enough to really appreciate the custom. Some of my best memories are of the long two- to three-hour lunches we took there. My children were born in Venezuela. The school they attended was within walking distance, so they got to come home for lunch. When they were in preschool, we always had a nap.

Now, businesses are too hurried, schools are too hurried, parents are too hurried, spouses are too hurried, and children are too hurried. Everyone is time deprived. The problem is everywhere! What are we to do?

THE WAY IT CAN BE

What God intended for our good can be reclaimed through practicing the three principles from the Creation's garden: healthy eating, physical activity, and rest. These three principles and their practical application are not common practice, but they are common sense. This concept is not a diet. It is not an exercise routine. It is not psychotherapy. These principles are guides for healthy living with the emphasis on *living*. The most exciting part is that scientific evidence is beginning to prove that these principles really are the basis of health and wellness.

Healthy Eating
For healthy eating, choose the following:

- Whole, unprocessed foods
- 100% whole grains and cereals
- Natural unrefined plant oils and no trans fats
- Organic meats and dairy products
- Locally grown fruits and vegetables when possible
- Water (about eight glasses per day)
- Breakfast to start the day
- Healthy snacks and desserts
- Nutrient-dense foods, or power foods, daily
- Moderate portions (no bigger than a deck of cards or a tennis ball)

Most important: Realize that all natural foods are good foods...when eaten in moderation!

God's abundant provision for Adam and Eve was repeated in His promise to the children of Israel in Deuteronomy 8:7–9: *"For the LORD your God is bringing you into a good land—a land with streams and pools of water, with springs flowing in the valleys and hills; a land with wheat and barley, vines and fig trees, pomegranates, olive oil and honey; a land where bread will not be scarce and you will lack nothing."*

If you have visited the Caribbean, Latin America, France, Italy, Spain, Greece, Asia, the South Pacific, or any other place where shopping for fresh food daily is the norm, then you have experienced the joy of seeing whole foods at their best. Having lived in Latin America for more than a decade, I truly miss this part of everyday living. I could spend hours going from one vendor to the next, touching, smelling, squeezing (being careful, of course), and tasting, just spellbound at the sights. Such memories steer my mind to the abundance of the Creation's garden, the promised land, paradise—fresh whole foods as far as you can see. Not just produce, but meat, poultry, eggs, seafood, legumes, nuts, yogurt, and cheeses. I can still smell the freshly baked bread and the roasting coffee beans in the markets of Venezuela and Costa Rica. I can taste the freshly squeezed tangerine juice—my favorite! I can see the purple pineapples (yes, purple), the blue-tinted eggs (from the grass the hens ate), and the freshly hung cheeses. I relish these memories; however, I do try to forget the flies!

In *Made for Paradise*, you will learn how to decide what to choose, how to choose it, and how to best enjoy it. You will discover the amazing relationship of whole fresh foods to health and wellness, just as God intended. We will take a look at the health benefits of natural foods, which we have all but abandoned in this country over the last century, and the health risks of processed foods that have been developed. We will look at methods of healthy food preparation, preservation, and presentation. We will see how to best estimate moderate portion sizes and value food quality over quantity—taste first! You will learn to appreciate the health benefits of water, God's original beverage and a blessing most of us take for granted. You will learn not only how to eat in, but also how to eat out with common sense—it's easier than you think!

With globalization, most Americans are beginning to appreciate many new tastes from around the world. Many of our most "American" foods are really adaptations of foreign foods. Hot dogs, pizza, doughnuts—all these have come into favor thanks to our melting pot! Variety is the spice of life (and food). The more variety, the more nutrients, the more colors, the more tastes. In this book, you will meet lots of new foods that I hope you will try. We also revisit traditional favorites and comfort foods. The delights are there for the taking. You'll be surprised what your taste buds just might discover—but in moderation, of course!

Physical Activity
For physical activity/exercise, choose the following:

- Common chores
- Sports activities
- Aerobic activity (intentional)
- Flexibility exercises
- Strength or resistance exercises
- Added daily activity for 10,000 steps

Most important: Just get moving!

So really, when were the good old days? When we all did manual labor? I don't think so! It does make sense, however, that modern conveniences and changes like car ownership, modern appliances, processed and convenience foods, TVs, computers, video games, sedentary occupations, elevators, escalators, urbanization, loss of sidewalks, lack of safety in neighborhoods, and a million other realities of modern life have contributed to the lack of physical activity in most American lifestyles. Just think of all the energy burned by chopping wood, fetching water from a well, washing clothes and hanging them by hand, plowing, planting, tending the crops, harvesting, and tending animals. It makes me tired just thinking about it, but all this was just part of a day's work. No wonder our great-grandparents ate bacon, eggs, pancakes, and biscuits and gravy and drank whole milk right from the cow—they needed the calories for their work.

I don't think most of us want to go back to days quite that good (except for maybe the breakfast), but common sense physical activities are all around us if we just think about it a little. *Made for Paradise* will give you ideas for burning calories through normal household activities, sports and recreation, walking, running, flexibility exercises, and strengthening/resistance exercises. You may choose any physical activity/exercise that floats your boat; you just have to get moving. We will talk a lot about walking and how to maximize this common sense way to burn energy. We will even look at flexibility and strengthening exercises you can do if you are basically stationary. If you have your doctor's permission, you really have no excuse for not strengthening those muscles, no matter how old they are! Strengthening exercises build muscles, and muscles burn energy. It's that simple. That's what they were made for. You may just need to remind them! The more muscle you build, the more energy you burn, even when you are not active. What a deal!

Rest

For rest (prayer, meditation, relaxation, and sleep), choose the following:

- Prayer, meditation, and quiet time daily
- Reconnection with nature
- Quiet hobbies, like games, reading, or knitting
- Time daily with your significant other and family
- Adequate sleep

Most important: Take the time...to take time...for God, for yourself, for your family.

Stress has always been and will always be with us. Life happens, and with life comes fear, anxiety, anger, resentment—stress! Our body has a natural hormonal response to stress. These hormones get our body ready for a physical response known as fight-or-flight reaction. We don't have to fight tigers or wild bears most days, but, nevertheless, when things go bump in the night, the same hormones are released. Over time, chronic stress, such as work or school pressures, family conflicts, or money worries, can lead to psychological distress or physical damage or both. Acute stress, such as sudden trauma, can also be dangerous in certain situations. A growing body of scientific research links stress to emotional and physical problems, such as depression, heart disease, hypertension, stroke, impaired immune function, infertility, insulin resistance, memory loss, gastrointestinal difficulties, and other chronic diseases. Our hurried lives, including inadequate sleep, tip the scales on stress.

On the bright side, other researchers show that mental/spiritual meditation, relaxation, and sleep lower stress and the physical reactions to it. Our bodies are literally set to an internal clock regulated by the sunshine of day and the darkness of night that helps regulate body systems. We will see how sunshine and dark themselves are necessary for our body. And guess what: Research links healthy eating, physical activity, and rest to health! It makes sense that God, who created us for wholeness, would give us the essentials for healthy living from the beginning.

In *Made for Paradise,* we will rediscover how to slow down and smell the roses—or the soup simmering. We will look at the aspects of mental/spiritual meditation, relaxation, and sleep that can help us manage daily stress and hopefully reduce those factors that put us at further risk for chronic disease.

LET'S GO THERE!

In the chapters that follow, we will explore Creation's garden together. We will walk step-by-step through the basic but profound principles of healthy living that should be common practice every day:

- Healthy eating (taking in energy and nutrients)
  Genesis 1:27–29 and 2:7–9

- Physical activity (burning energy)
  Genesis 2:15

- Rest (meditation, relaxation, and sleep)
  Genesis 2:2–3 and 3:8

Until that wonderful day when believers live in the midst of God's restored paradise, we can only walk toward that kind of perfect wholeness.

God says of heaven in Amos 9:11–15 that He will restore the house of David and the people of Israel *"will rebuild the ruined cities and live in them. They will plant vineyards and drink their wine; they will make gardens and eat their fruit"* (v. 14). God will restore Israel to the New Jerusalem, and they will never again be uprooted from the land He gave to them.

In our heavenly home on each side of the river of the water of life, there will be trees of life bearing fruit every month. The fruit of the trees will be for food and the leaves of the trees will be for the healing of the nations. The Lord God will be our light and we will serve Him, praise Him, and honor Him forever and ever (Revelation 22:1–5). *"No eye has seen, no ear has heard, no mind has conceived what God has prepared for those who love him"* (1 Corinthians 2:9, referring to Isaiah 64:4). There is no way we finite humans can get our brains around the paradise that God has waiting for us. I do think that in the meantime, however, He doesn't want us to miss the closest thing to heaven on earth!

Our bodies function as they should if we adhere to the Manufacturer's instructions. We celebrate His world and enjoy His blessing of healthy eating every time we sit down to savor a bite of His glorious bounty! We honor Him with the service of our daily physical activity, work, and living. We rest in Him literally and spiritually to renew our strength. May God give us the desire, the wisdom, and the common sense to choose to live in the paradise He created for us.

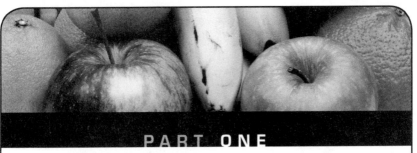

PART ONE
HEALTHY EATING

God saw all that he had made,
and it was very good.
—Genesis 1:31

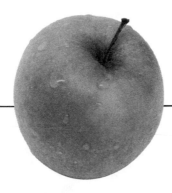

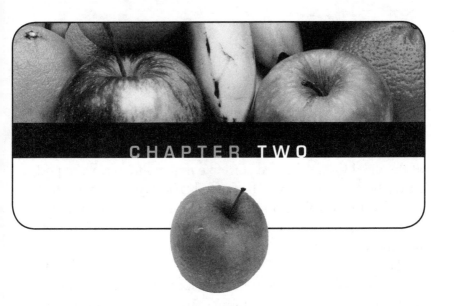

CHAPTER TWO

WHOLE FOODS REIGN

●

*[The LORD] makes grass grow for the cattle, and plants for man to cultivate—
bringing forth food from the earth: wine that gladdens the heart of man,
oil to make his face shine, and bread that sustains his heart.*
—Psalm 104:14–15

BOTH the Old Testament and the New Testament are rich with references to the grains, nuts, seeds, legumes, fruits, and vegetables native to the Middle East. From Creation's garden through thousands of years of history, civilizations have depended on gathering and preparing locally grown whole plant food. Eventually, the cultivation of crops evolved in the Middle East—first, grains like wheat and barley; then pistachios, almonds, grapes, dates, figs, melons, pomegranates, beans, peas, garlic, onions, cucumbers, herbs, and olives.

The term *whole foods* simply means foods as close to their natural state as possible—best if fresh and locally grown! What is more heavenly on a late August afternoon than a watermelon right out of the patch? Or a fresh, ripe, red tomato pulled right off the vine! Or just-husked corn five minutes from stalk to pot! Throughout history, whole fresh foods had been eaten in their natural state until about 150 years ago. If not eaten raw or freshly cooked, foods had been preserved by drying, salting, smoking, fermenting, or curdling.

The Industrial Revolution brought with it the ability to preserve food for food safety, but also for convenience and mass production. The mass production of processed and convenience foods has changed not only *how* we eat, but *what* we eat. Locally grown produce has been replaced with every food imaginable— available at our fingertips, both in and out of season. We may be able to eat peaches in February, but the nutritional value and taste of the natural whole food has been compromised by early harvest and/or storage. This is not to say that we should never eat produce from California, Florida, Chile, or Spain that is out of season in our home state, but the taste and nutritional value of locally grown produce will usually be superior, and by purchasing local produce, you will be supporting small farmers and your local economy.

For me, one of the greatest differences in living in Latin America as opposed to the United States was the experience of grocery shopping. What we take for granted as we walk through the aisles of our local grocery stores is the *convenience* of shopping for food. What we are missing is the *adventure* of shopping for food. The purchase of groceries is a full-time job in the Third World and traditional, nonindustrialized countries. You get your bread from the bakery—right out of the oven! You get your meat from the butcher. You get your vegetables from the vegetable market. You get your fruit from the fruit market. You get staples, such as milk, rice, coffee, tea, and flour, from the neighborhood store if you are lucky. In some countries, you do this every day. The trade-off for convenience is *freshness*. Everything is fresh—sometimes too fresh (like meat). Since there are no frozen foods or convenience foods, all recipes are made from scratch—time consuming, but wonderful.

One of the best resources I have found for learning to prepare whole foods from scratch is the *More-with-Less Cookbook* by Doris Longacre. This classic cookbook celebrated its twenty-fifth anniversary in 2000. The idea is that we can make more with less as we turn to basic simple recipes made from fresh whole foods; these useful cookbooks promote this idea:

- *More-with-Less Cookbook* by Doris J. Longacre
- *The Whole Foods Market Cookbook* by Steve Petusevsky
- *The Organic Food Guide* by Steve Meyerowitz

As we walk through the Creation's garden together in the pages of this book, we will look at practical, everyday, *yummy* ways to bring whole foods to your table.

FOOD STARTS WITH FARMING

For many generations, traditional American farmers—from George Washington and Thomas Jefferson to our own grandparents—have worked to protect the land and the quality of rural life. That doesn't mean that they were not innovative. On the contrary, Jefferson, for instance, was always testing new crops and varieties and farming methods that were best suited to the land and the needs of people. These concepts included taking care of the lands that were being farmed. This was necessary and expected. This was sustainable agriculture—farming that maintained the environment and used renewable natural resources in a manner that would enrich farmlands, not exhaust them.

After the end of World War II, the development and use of chemical pesticides and fertilizers began to increase crop yields tremendously. About the same time, industrialized one-crop farms owned by large corporations began to increase and receive subsidies from the federal government. Many small farmers just could not compete. Although these large one-crop megafarms have helped lower food prices in the United States, they have also contributed to the lowering of nutrients in the soil and in the crops. This makes the use of more chemical fertilizers necessary. The growing of monocrops increases the use of pesticides, and more pesticides deplete the soil of more nutrients.

Chemical pesticides and fertilizers not only deplete crops of nutrients, but chemical runoffs also contaminate ground water. Every year during the summer, a large part (the size of New Jersey!) of the Gulf of Mexico at the mouth of the Mississippi River becomes uninhabitable by sea life. Agricultural runoff from large megafarms along the river, as well as other industrial waste from large factory farms for animals, like cattle, pork, and poultry, deplete the oxygen in the water. This "dead zone" and many others around the US have been growing for more than 30 years. Increased use of chemicals on farms over the last few decades has not only contributed to the general rise in the incidence of cancers in the United States, but farm workers themselves have the highest rates of chemically induced illnesses of any group. In 1970, after almost 30 years of chemical use on farms and in other industries, the US Environmental Protection Agency was created to help regulate chemical contamination of our land and water and, thus, the food chain. This attempt at regulation came after research began to show the detrimental effects of chemicals on every aspect of the environment. In 1972, DDT, the first modern pesticide, was banned. Today, DDT residue can still be found in our foods! Many pesticides and fertilizers banned in the US are still being sold overseas. That means that imported produce must be cleaned thoroughly, as should US produce that is most vulnerable to residue. (Washing techniques will be discussed in a later chapter.)

The food chain has also been affected by a change in the way animals are raised. Grass feeding of animals was common in this country until about 85 years ago, when factory farming of animals began as a means of increasing production. With factory farming, the animals are raised in confined spaces and given antibiotics, hormones, and other chemicals to enhance productivity.

Farmers and consumers, both, are waking up. Organic foods—foods produced according to organic standards (for example, crops grown without the use of conventional pesticides or artificial fertilizers and animals reared without the routine use of antibiotics, hormones, or other chemicals)—which were thought of as "hippie food" in the 1960s and 1970s, began a comeback in the 1980s and 1990s. Increasingly, more farmers are returning to natural sustainable farm and dairy methods, including organics. Also, more consumers are demanding organic and natural foods for health reasons—and taste! The vitamins and other nutrients carried especially in the fat of grass-fed animals (meat, milk, and egg yolks) are essential for healthy eating. The concept of locally produced foods from small multicrop farms, gardens, and dairies is gradually coming back—hopefully to your neighborhood!

Community supported agriculture (CSA)—similar to what many call truck farming—is a partnership of local farmers and consumers. Consumers purchase a share of each season's harvest; this covers the farms' operating budgets. Then the members divide the bounty of fresh, local produce. CSA brings back the direct connection between the farmer, the land he farms, the food he produces, and the people who eat that food. Sustainable, community supported agriculture that includes organic farming is the future of farming in this country, as well as its history.

Another way to support sustainable agriculture is to look for the Fair Trade Certified™ label on food products. Fair Trade is a market-based approach to sustainable development that helps family farmers in developing countries gain direct access to international markets. When they learn how to market their own harvests, Fair Trade farmers are able to receive a fair price for their products. This leads to higher family living standards, thriving com-munities, and more sustainable farming practices. Fair Trade enables farming families to take care of themselves—without

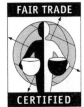

Look for this label.

developing a dependency on foreign aid. Look for the Fair Trade Certified™ label on coffee, tea, cocoa, chocolate, sugar, honey, fruit juice, and fresh fruit.

WHOLE—THE WAY GOD MADE FOOD

Let me explain more to you about the benefits of whole foods. It's amazing! We really are meant to eat foods as God created them. Recent scientific research has given the medical community the body of knowledge it needed to prove that what our mothers said was true—we need to eat our vegetables and fruits. Advancements in analysis of foods has allowed us to see beyond the value of traditional vitamins and minerals, which were discovered in the last century, to understand the literally thousands of food compounds in whole foods now known as phytochemicals. Phytochemicals work as antioxidants in our bodies just as do vitamin C, vitamin E, beta-carotene, and the mineral selenium. Antioxidants are compounds in our foods that protect our cells against damage from oxygen and reduce our risk of chronic diseases, such as heart disease and cancer. Antioxidants and phytochemicals are found most abundantly in whole foods, such as fruits, vegetables, herbs, whole grains, nuts, seeds, and legumes. The most important principle about health benefits from these foods, however, is that whole foods contain the most phytochemicals. All of these compounds, including vitamins, minerals, and phytochemicals, act synergistically as we consume whole foods on a daily basis. Single nutrient supplements may give health benefits to those with specific medical conditions, but, in general, the consumption of whole natural foods the way God made them gives us the most benefit.

The whole foods concept also includes meat, poultry, eggs, and dairy products in their most natural states. This means it is better to use organic products from grass-fed animals. Natural compounds in these animal foods, which are processed as little as possible, give us the most health benefits from sources that are not fully understood, just as those in natural whole plants. These nutrients will be discussed in coming chapters.

Should we be surprised that the nutrients we need for healthy bodies (that God made) come from natural foods (that God made)? *Hello!* From the ability to isolate specific food components, we are learning that it is the working together of all of these nutritional components that gives the greatest protection against disease. These known nutritional compounds (vitamins, minerals, and phytochemicals) and unknown ones, of which there are thousands, are all found only in whole foods. How convenient! In addition to these compounds working together *in* specific foods, there may also be a synergy of nutritional compounds interacting *between* these foods and others in the diet. The more variety, the better! It may be more important to evaluate the pattern of foods we eat than what specific foods we eat. Clearly, whole foods work together in complex ways for our overall health and well-being— ways that we are just now discovering. This is another example of our Maker providing *from the beginning* for all of His creation.

DON'T MESS WITH A GOOD THING!

The opposite of a whole food is a refined or processed food. The more refined or processed a food is, the less it resembles the original food, the more original nutrients are lost, and the longer the ingredient list on the food label becomes. Some nutrients that are destroyed in the refining and processing of foods may be added back; but since we don't know all the nutritional compounds in a food, they cannot *all* be added back! Most refined grain products add thiamin, riboflavin, niacin, and iron back, but other vitamins, minerals, and phytochemicals are lost.

Processing of grains began as early as the fourth century B.C. White bread was a status symbol, with dark bread relegated to peasants, athletes, and slaves. However, even that far back in history, some people—including Hippocrates—insisted that whole grains were better for health. B vitamins were first discovered in the husks of rice in the early twentieth century. We now know that valuable vitamins and minerals and other nutrients lurk just underneath the surface of the bran or husk of all grain and under the peels of fruits and vegetables!

Processing of milk (pasteurization and homogenization) destroys the natural properties of raw milk and milk products. God put animal fat with animal meat for a reason. Could raw milk and animal meat actually be good for us?

Research shows that whole foods rich in natural vitamins, minerals, antioxidants, phytochemicals, proteins, and fats are what make our body, and especially our brain, function as it should. Some snack foods, fast foods, and manufactured foods do not. We will explore these and other examples of the nutritional benefits of whole natural foods. The power of whole foods as God created them is amazing!

Since whole foods are so much better for our bodies, you may need some guidelines for retaining the nutrients in whole foods. So here we go:

- Select produce with care; look for any damage.

- Eat produce as soon as possible. If storage is necessary, be sure it is airtight.

- When storing produce, avoid excessive heat, light, air (especially dry air), or moisture. Don't allow the produce to be cut or bruised. If produce is stored at room temperature, avoid direct sunlight.

- Wash fruits and vegetables just before eating or preparing.

- If possible, eat vegetables and fruits whole, including skin, husks, membranes, and seeds.

- If cooking vegetables and fruits, steam, microwave, or stir-fry them.

- If boiling vegetables and fruits, many vitamins and minerals will remain in the water, so use it!

- Reheat leftover produce in a microwave, if possible, for quick heating.

- Store virgin olive oil in a dark, cool place.

- Store whole grains and cereals in the freezer if not using right away.

- Choose organic grass-fed meat and poultry (and eggs of the same) when possible.

- When possible, choose organic milk and milk products, including butter, from grass-fed cows.

Since we can't turn back the clock, it is likely that we will always be eating and cooking with some processed food products. However, we can consciously choose whole natural foods and processed foods with the smallest ingredient list on the label. Food labels must include a list of ingredients in descending order by weight. Look for a whole food listed first. Also beware of hydrogenated fats and sugars near the beginning of the list: hydrogenated or partially hydrogenated fats, high-fructose corn syrup, sucrose, maltose, dextrose, hydrolyzed starch, invert sugar, or molasses.

Artificial food additives are another issue related to refined and processed foods. Chemicals are added to processed foods to improve shelf life, storage time, flavor, nutritional value, and attractiveness and to make food more convenient and easy to prepare. Again, the more ingredients listed on the food label, the more additives are probably in that food product. Common sense should tell us that the more artificial ingredients we consume, the more health risks we are taking. Various food additives have been implicated in increasing the risks of allergies, asthma, behavioral changes, impaired immune function, and cancer—to name a few.

If this is a risk for adults, it is an even greater risk for children. Foods that contain chemicals in amounts that would not be harmful to adults might be dangerous for children, because the chemicals could accumulate more quickly due to their small size. We simply do not know what effect decades of consuming food additives and chemicals will have on our children. Other additives that end up in meat, poultry, eggs, and dairy products from antibiotics and hormones given to animals may also be worrisome. The issues of antibiotic and hormone residues in these foods will be discussed in later chapters. It can be really scary!

Read food labels! Additives to limit or avoid include artificial colors and flavors, artificial sweeteners and fats, nitrites and nitrates, sulfites, and preservatives (BHA, BHT, EDTA, etc.). **Remember: If it is hard to pronounce, it is probably artificial!**

GENETIC ENGINEERING

Remember how we all learned about genetic engineering from the news stories on cloning? Well, it is now possible to genetically modify foods. Genetically modified foods or organisms (GMOs) are another departure from nature that the United States has yet to tackle in earnest. Historically, food crops and animals have been bred naturally to improve the yield, taste, health, and hardiness of food sources. This traditional breeding can only take place between closely related species.

With genetic engineering, genetic information from one species can be inserted into an organism of another species, or bacterial and viral genes can be put into plants, as is done with most genetically engineered foods. Genetic engineering allows DNA to be moved between unrelated organisms.

In some countries, such as the United Kingdom, food producers must indicate on labels whether the food contains genetically modified ingredients. This, however, is not the case in the United States, where many common grocery items now contain genetically modified ingredients but are not labeled as such.

Below is a list of foods that may contain genetically modified organisms (GMOs):

- **Vegetable oils:** canola (rape/rapeseed), margarine, cotton, soy, flax, or corn oil labeled as vegetable
- **Produce:** tomatoes, soybeans, corn, squash, papaya, cassava, coffee beans
- **Soybeans:** processed foods, hydrolyzed vegetable protein, textured vegetable protein, vegetable protein extract, soy protein, lecithin emulsifier, tofu, tempeh, soy sauce, soy fiber
- **Corn:** corn starch, glucose syrup, starch, modified starch, thickener, corn flour, corn flakes, cereals, snack foods
- **Potatoes:** potato starch and flour

GENETICALLY MODIFIED SEEDS

Genetically modified seeds are another problem. Genetically modified seeds and plants often have changes in genes that code for certain proteins to give the plant some unique benefit. Benefits include the ability to produce more chemicals to fight infection, pests, or frosts; resistance to a pesticide or herbicide used to kill other plants; higher production of a particular type of amino acid or fat; or other benefit.

One kind of seed, called first generation hybrids (F1 hybrids), has been hand-pollinated. F1 hybrids are patented, genetically identical within food types, and sold by multinational seed companies.

A second kind of seed is genetically engineered. These seeds are fast contaminating the global seed supply on a wholesale level and threatening the purity of seeds everywhere. The DNA of the plant has been changed. A cold-water fish gene could be spliced into a tomato to make the plant more resistant to frost, for example.

A third kind of seed is called heirloom or open pollinated. These are seeds that have been passed on from generation to generation. Heirloom seeds offer us genetic diversity that is highlighted by a wide range of colors, textures, shapes, and flavors. It is because of this genetic diversity that heirloom seeds are so vital. Not only are growers protecting genetic diversity, but they are also preserving history. Some heirloom seeds can be traced back more than a hundred years. Preserving the cycle of growing and saving seed continues the cycle of God's creation and allows us to share a piece of history with family and friends. Here are some Web sites for seed-saving organizations:

- *www.seedsavers.org*
- *www.nativeseeds.org*
- *www.southernexposure.com*
- *www.seedsofchange.com*
- *www.seedman.com*
- *www.heirloomseeds.com*

RESISTANCE TO GMO FOOD

In Europe, resistance to GMO food is greater than ever. GMO food is rejected by the majority of European food brands, retailers, and consumers. GMO crops are illegal in Switzerland and prohibited by 175 regional governments and by over 4,500 local authorities and smaller areas in 22 European Union (EU) countries because of their health, environmental, and economic risks. Most European countries started banning GMOs as early as 1999. The debate over GMOs will probably continue overseas and eventually gear up in the United States. One of the only states so far to vote on the ban of GMO food is California. Since that state led the nation in the revival of organic foods, it seems natural that the GMO debate in the US would begin in earnest on the West Coast.

Genetic engineering raises a lot of issues. Some see it as beneficial—for instance, as a way to combat hunger in nations with low food production—and some see it as harmful. Probably we aren't capable right now of foreseeing the long-term effects of GMOs.

However, it seems to me like a good idea to leave God's creation alone! In the Book of Job, chapter 28, Job said, "*Where then does wisdom come from? Where does understanding dwell?... God understands the way to it and he alone knows where it dwells, for he views the ends of the earth and sees everything under the heavens*" (vv. 20, 23–24). Proverbs 14:12 states, "*There is a way that seems right to a man, but in the end it leads to death.*" The potential benefits of GMO crops should not be ignored, but the risks should be carefully weighed. As Christians, we respect the fact that God gave humanity the responsibility to guard, care for, and tend to God's creation. We must require an evaluation of the potential direct and indirect long-term effects of GMO crops on our health and the environment.

FINDING A WAY BACK

With that said, should we avoid all processed foods, GMO foods, and food additives? Of course not! That would be nearly impossible for most of us. However, choosing whole natural foods for most meals and as a way of life gives us the flexibility to also use processed foods in moderation.

The only way to find our way back to whole natural foods is to demand them. We as consumers can be powerful people when we use the influence of our wallets! The demand for whole natural foods in some areas of the US is beginning to make a difference. Look for these helpful references:

- *The Whole Foods Market Cookbook* by Steve Petusevsky
- *Foods That Fight Disease* by Laurie Deutsch Mozian
- *The Real Food Revival* by Sherri Vinton and Ann Espuelas
- *Real Food: What to Eat and Why* by Nina Planck

The first step is to become aware of what you and your family are currently eating. Begin to choose more locally grown, natural products (organic when possible). Find retailers in your area that stock whole, natural foods. Look for the Fair Trade label. Ask your grocer to supply a bigger local organic food section in his store. Try looking for natural whole foods online, and find local organic dairies and farms (*www.foodroutes.org* or *www.localharvest.org*). You might be surprised what gems you find in your community. Support your local farmers market, and **remember to buy fresh and buy local!**

Even if we do eat whole natural foods, we still need to know more specifically what to eat for healthy living and how much of it. God gave us all the foods we enjoy, but are they all created equal? Not really! *Dietary Guidelines for Americans 2005*, published jointly by the Department of Health and Human Services (HHS) and the Department of Agriculture (USDA), and the USDA's Food Guide Pyramid, revised in 2005, give us a good start. These guidelines are a great way to estimate the variety and quantity of foods that each age group needs to eat every day. We will be referring to and tweaking the *Dietary Guidelines* (*www.healthierus.gov/dietaryguidelines*) and Food Guide Pyramid (*www.mypyramid.gov*) as we move through *Made for Paradise*. The basic principles of healthy eating can be summarized into three easy-to-remember points: (1) Eat a variety of foods. (2) Know what you are eating. (3) No portion of any food should be bigger than a deck of cards or a tennis ball.

The average American eats more food at one sitting that most people from other countries eat in a day! It's sad, but true. Miss Piggy is quoted as saying, "Never eat more than you can lift." Before following that advice, consider the source. Moses more wisely said, *"You may be sure that your sin will find you out"* (Numbers 32:23). And gluttony is surely a sin! More about that later.

REMEMBER!

There are three basic principles of healthy eating:

- Eat a variety of whole foods, choosing local and organic when possible.
- Read food labels.
- Limit portion sizes.

Remember: Make whole foods reign!

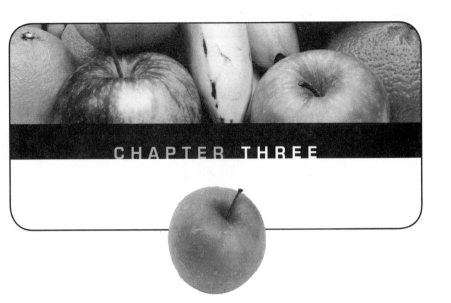

CHAPTER THREE

CARBOHYDRATES: TRUTH AND CONSEQUENCES

———————•———————

[Jesus] said to them, "When you pray, say: 'Father, hallowed be your name, your kingdom come. Give us each day our daily bread. Forgive us our sins, for we also forgive everyone who sins against us. And lead us not into temptation.'"
—Luke 11:2–4

HUMANS have considered whole grains and cereals as dietary staples throughout recorded history. Barley played an important role in ancient culture as a staple grain as well as an important food for athletes, who attributed much of their strength to their barley-containing training diets. Gladiators were actually known as "eaters of barley." When God was leading the Israelites through the desert from Egypt, they were promised a land of wheat and barley, where bread would not be scarce (Deuteronomy 8:8–9). Current research is rediscovering the many health benefits of eating whole grains and legumes; those benefits include reduced risk of obesity and reduced risk of certain diseases, such as heart disease, cancer, and diverticular disease (pockets in the colon). Other research has focused on the protective effects of phytochemicals (plant chemicals) in whole grains and cereals. These health benefits are found in grains and cereals that have not been processed or refined: whole wheat, bulgur, barley, oats, corn, millet, rye, buckwheat, quinoa, spelt, amaranth, brown rice, and many more!

Kernels of whole grains, such as wheat, barley, oats, rye, corn, and rice, consist of three major parts: the bran or outer layer, which contains B vitamins and minerals; the endosperm, or inner starch; and the germ, which contains the grain oil and fat-soluble vitamins and minerals. The bran and germ are also rich sources of antioxidants, including vitamin E and selenium, as well as phytochemicals. When grains are processed or refined, both the bran and the germ are removed. In enriched breads and cereals, some of the B vitamins and iron are added back, but the protective effects of the whole grain are lost.

Many of the health benefits in whole grains and cereals are found in the dietary fibers of the bran. Dietary fiber refers to carbohydrates that our systems cannot digest. Dietary fiber is found in all plants that are eaten for food, including grains, legumes, fruits, and vegetables. Dietary fiber in these foods is a mix of two kinds of fiber: soluble fiber, found in abundance in oatmeal, nuts, seeds, legumes (beans, peas, and lentils), and many fruits; and insoluble fiber, found mostly in the bran of whole grains, seeds, and many vegetables. Soluble and insoluble fibers contain powerful phytochemicals that protect against heart disease and breast, prostate, and colon cancers. Since the most health-protective benefits come when foods are eaten whole, this is even more reason to eat foods as close to their natural state as possible.

Another source of carbohydrate that acts like dietary fiber in the digestive system is resistant starch. Resistant starches are abundant in unprocessed whole grains and cereals, durum wheat (semolina) pasta, potatoes, bananas, and especially beans and peas. Dietary fiber and resistant starches play a very important role in the prevention of obesity and in decreasing the risk for diseases that develop from obesity.

WHAT IS THE PROBLEM?

Research in the last few years has found relationship between carbohydrate absorption, obesity, heart disease, and type 2 diabetes. Some have called this relationship the metabolic syndrome. This syndrome is characterized by a group of conditions that includes the following four:

- Central obesity (fatty tissue in and around the abdomen)
- High blood cholesterol levels
- Increased blood pressure
- Insulin resistance or glucose intolerance (condition in which blood cannot regulate blood sugar properly)

Researchers now know that the majority of these symptoms begin with obesity, which impairs insulin's ability to process blood sugar. As a result, the body stores excess sugar calories as fat in the abdominal region. This excess fat increases risk for high blood pressure, heart disease, and type 2 diabetes. This phenomenon is called glycemic response and is a measure of food's ability to elevate blood sugar.

All food is digested into the simple sugar glucose. After a meal, the faster glucose is absorbed into the blood, the more insulin is secreted from the pancreas to take the glucose from the blood into the organs. Too much insulin in the blood makes blood sugar drop too far, signaling more hunger. Elevated secretion of insulin in response to high blood glucose can eventually lead to obesity, which may lead to insulin resistance, high blood pressure, and type 2 diabetes. Men, in general, tend to gain weight in their midsections, and after the hormonal changes of menopause, so do women. In the last 20 years, obesity and type 2 diabetes have doubled in the United States.

In 2002, the Centers for Disease Control (CDC) reported that more than one in five Americans have metabolic syndrome. A recent report by the CDC said that in the near future, obesity would probably become the leading preventable cause of death in the US, overtaking heart disease.

WHAT IS THE SOLUTION?

In addition to increasing activity and exercise, one key to preventing metabolic syndrome is to slow down carbohydrate digestion and break the cycle of insulin spikes, hunger, and weight gain. Choosing high-fiber whole grains, legumes, vegetables, and fruits as the bulk of our food and avoiding refined carbohydrates like sugar and highly processed grains and cereals are ways of doing this. So for better health, choose the following:

- Whole grain breads, cereals, pasta, and rice for dietary fiber
- Pasta from durum wheat (semolina)
- A wide variety of beans and peas for dietary fiber and resistant starch
- Added dietary fiber, like All-Bran (add to recipes)
- Good fats, such as olive and peanut oils, to slow digestion
- Moderate amounts of protein at meals to slow digestion
- Acids like lemon juice and vinegar to slow digestion

These combinations of foods can slow down glycemic response, which will gradually even out the insulin spikes and carbohydrate cravings that accompany the eating of refined foods. The same dietary principles apply for persons who want to lower intake of refined carbohydrates, persons with insulin resistance or prediabetes, and others who are already diagnosed with diabetes. If a person already has diabetes, it is important to work with a doctor or a registered dietitian (RD) to regulate his or her meal pattern with any diabetic medication being taking.

In addition to choosing more whole grain and cereal products, it is also important to limit the use of refined sugars in our everyday diet. Thirty years ago, most of the sugar in the American diet came from sugarcane or sugar beets. Now, much of the sugar in processed foods comes from high-fructose corn syrup (HFCS). The increase of its use from the 1970s until today is well over 1,000%. This syrup is not only cheaper for manufacturers to use, but much sweeter. Look for HFCS in such products as soft drinks, sweet tea (for you southerners), fruit juices, baked goods, salad dressings, canned fruits, dairy products, nondairy creamers, cookies, gum, jams, and jellies. Needless to say, the overconsumption of all refined carbohydrates should be guarded against, but especially that of HFCS in children and teens.

The variety of whole grain products available in our grocery stores has grown by leaps and bounds, partly due to the globalization of our palates and also to the revitalization of historical grains and cereals long forgotten. Whole grains contain the entire grain kernel—bran, germ, and endosperm. Examples include whole wheat flour, bulgur (cracked wheat), oatmeal, rye, whole cornmeal, brown rice, buckwheat, amaranth, millet, quinoa, sorghum, kamut, spelt, teff, and triticale. Never heard of some of these? Take time to browse through your baking and cereal aisle at the grocery to identify products that contain familiar and some not-so-familiar grains and cereals. You can read more about all of these products at the Whole Grains Council Web site (*www.wholegrainscouncil.org*). You may want to check out *The New Book of Whole Grains* by Marlene Anne Bumgarner. Experiment and have fun!

RICE AND PASTA

Since rice feeds half the population of the world—all of Asia—special mention must be made of this important staple. Brown rice is more nutritious than polished or semipolished white rice, of course, but many varieties of rice are grown and eaten in Asia. Many people and organizations consider rice to be the world's most important food. It is second only to wheat as the most widely cultivated cereal in the world. In much of Asia, rice is so central to the culture that the word is almost synonymous with food. In Chinese, the *"daily bread"* line in the Lord's Prayer is translated as *"give us this day our daily rice,"* and a Japanese proverb states, "A meal without rice is no meal." Grown in Asia for at least 10,000 years, rice has influenced the cultures and lives of billions of people. Throughout this vast region, rice still dominates customs, beliefs, rituals, and celebrations. Rice is eaten at least three times a day, but it is combined with vegetables, fruit, nuts, tofu, fish, and maybe some meat.

Like rice, pasta is a food that has been eaten for thousands of years. It is a central ingredient in the Mediterranean meal pattern, which has been linked to health and longevity. The traditional Mediterranean diet delivers as much as 40% of total daily calories from fat—olive oil—yet the associated incidence of cardiovascular diseases is significantly decreased. Eating olive oil every day and fish a few times a week benefits the Mediterranean people by increasing important phytochemicals and fatty acids in their diet. They also eat grains (such as pasta), fruits, vegetables, legumes, and nuts and drink red wine to round out their healthy eating.

Although pasta can be made of whole wheat, it is usually made of refined durum or semolina wheat. Pasta is made from wheat with a very high content of protein that is digested in the body like whole grain, so don't let anyone tell you that pasta is not healthy!

A world of grains and cereals is out there to investigate, cook, and love. You may enjoy old favorites, but don't get stuck in a rut. If sandwiches are a daily mainstay of yours, try new whole grain breads, but remember that one serving is just one slice. If your favorite burger joint serves only low-fiber white buns, request 100% whole wheat or take your own (which I have been known to do, to my children's chagrin)!

The document *Dietary Guidelines for Americans 2005* suggests that most adults eat at least three servings (1 ounce each) of whole grain products and cereals a day. A 1-ounce serving equals one slice of bread, 1 cup of dry cereal, or ½ cup of cooked cereal or pasta. Refer to *www.mypyramid.gov* for more information about serving and portion sizes. **Remember: A rule of thumb is that no portion of any food should be bigger than a deck of cards or a tennis ball.**

READING LABELS IS A MUST

Look for 100% whole grain first in the ingredient list. Choose 100% whole grain stone ground when possible. No machinery has yet been developed that grinds grains into flours, cereals, meals, and mixes quite as well as the millstones used since Roman times. Millstones grind the bran, endosperm, and germ in a cool, natural way. This cool stone-grinding process preserves valuable nutrients that would be lost by conventional milling. You can find 100% stone-ground products in many varieties of grains.

Look for 100% whole grain breads, cereals, and baked goods that contain at least 3 grams of dietary fiber per serving and have the Whole Grain™ stamp.

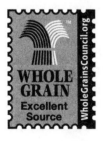

Whole Grain™ Stamps are a trademark of Oldways Preservation Trust and the Whole Grains Council. Courtesy of Oldways Preservation Trust and the Whole Grains Council. *www.wholegrainscouncil.org* and *www.oldwayspt.org*.

According to the Whole Grains Council, a true whole grain product will have 2 to 5 grams of dietary fiber. Cereal companies and bakery manufacturers have heard the consumer's demand for more products with whole grain. It is possible to find cereals that contain up to 14 grams of dietary fiber in just one serving! However, it is important to read the label carefully. Lean toward the products with more than 3 grams of dietary fiber and a daily value of 20% or more. Compare the content of dietary fiber and the sugar content to make a final decision.

Whole grain flours may be used in most recipes that call for white flour: substitute whole wheat flour for about one-fourth of the white flour, or substitute whole wheat pastry flour, cup for cup, for the white flour. Experiment with all the varieties of whole grain flours available. Resources and recipes may be found at *www.bobsredmill.com* and *www.kingarthurflour.com*.

VERSATILE GRANOLA

Granola is a versatile cereal. It's great for backpacking, snacks, and quick breakfasts. Homemade granolas are easy to make. They should be stored in tightly sealed containers in a cool area. Try granola toppings on your favorite fruit or on ice cream.

If there is one secret to making a good granola, it is mixing the ingredients well. Combine all of the liquid ingredients first. Briefly heating (using low temperature) honey or molasses and oil liquefies the mixture for better mixing. Slowly drizzle the liquid over the dry mixture. Stir it well to ensure even coverage.

Most recipes for granolas recommend baking the grain mixture in a warm oven (250°F to 300°F). This produces a crunchy granola with a lightly toasted, nutty flavor. Baking, however, is not essential. Granola may also be dried. A dried granola is chewier, lighter tasting, and more digestible. Dried granolas are especially good for using in other recipes. For a roasted flavor, lightly toast grains before mixing. When baking granolas, add any dried fruit after removing mixture from the oven. If you are drying the granola, the fruit may be added at any time. Granola ingredients include all kinds of good stuff: whole grains, such as rolled oats, wheat, rye, barley, and other whole grain flakes; a variety of nuts and seeds; dried fruits; honey or molasses; cinnamon, nutmeg, and other spices; and vanilla. One older but great book for granola recipes is *Granola Madness: The Ultimate Granola Cookbook* by Donna Wallstin and Katherine Dieter. Recipe Web sites also have lots of granola and trail mix ideas.

REMEMBER!

Add whole grains to your daily intake.

- Count all the dietary fiber from whole grains and cereals, legumes, vegetables, and fruits to be sure you eat about 25 to 30 grams per day.

- Choose grain and cereal products labeled as 100% whole grain, and look for the Whole Grain™ stamp.

- Choose 100% whole grain stone ground when possible.

- Choose grain and cereal products that contain at least 3 grams of dietary fiber.

- Add extra oat, wheat, or rice bran and wheat germ to cereal and casseroles.

- Make your own healthy granola and trail mix.

- Add oats to fruit desserts.

- Pop your own popcorn in light unrefined olive, sesame, or peanut oil. (I add a little butter to the oil.)

- Use whole wheat pastry flour instead of white flour in cakes, cookies, quick breads, and pastries.

- Use white whole wheat flour if your family does not like brown bread.

- Try using a cereal or grain that is unfamiliar to you.

- Make pasta or choose commercial pasta made with 100% durum (semolina) wheat flour.

- Avoid grain and cereal products that contain high-fructose corn syrup (HFCS).

Remember: Think 100% whole grains!

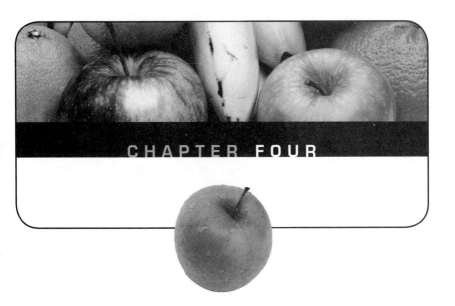

CHAPTER FOUR

WILL THE HEALTHY FATS PLEASE STAND UP?

———————•———————

*"I will give you the best of the land of Egypt
and you can enjoy the fat of the land."*
—Genesis 45:18

HEALTHY fats? Yes! Am I kidding? No!

For the last two decades, while Americans have purchased and eaten more and more fat-free and reduced-fat products, obesity in America has doubled. While these foods contain fewer calories from fat, they tend to have more calories from sugar and other refined carbohydrates—thus the same amount of calories or more.

Contrary to the low-fat, low-cholesterol diet recommendations of the last 20 years, research now shows that **it is the type of fat eaten that makes the difference in disease risk.** We are allowed some fat—in moderation. The idea is to substitute healthy fats for unhealthy fats. All fats have twice the number of calories per gram as do proteins or carbohydrates; however, some oils, such as olive, flaxseed, and fish oils, eaten in moderation, help protect against certain cancers and heart disease and help regulate blood sugar. Of course, too much animal fat is unhealthy, but the main culprits in increased disease risk are **refined and hydrogenated or even partially hydrogenated vegetable oils.** Virgin, naturally pressed, unrefined oils—the healthy fats—can be found at *www.spectrumorganics.com* and *www.tropicaltraditions.com*.

FAT AND CHOLESTEROL—WE NEED THEM

Actually, fat has many important functions in food as well as in the body. Fats give foods flavor and smooth texture, as well as extra calories! Food fats help slow the rate of digestion and give a feeling of satiety after eating. Several essential nutrients like essential fatty acids (found only in foods and not manufactured by the body) are soluble (or absorbed) only in fats. Omega-3 fatty acids are abundant in milk, milk products, and eggs from grass-fed animals. Fats act as carriers for the fat-soluble vitamins A, D, E, and K, which, in turn, are important for the absorption of many other nutrients in the body.

Cholesterol also has vital functions in our body, such as hormone formation, cell membrane structure, and production of vitamin D. Actually, dietary cholesterol found only in animal foods has very little relationship to the level of blood cholesterol in our bodies, since our liver also produces cholesterol. Dietary cholesterol from animal foods includes the cholesterol in meats, eggs, and shellfish. In fact, shellfish are rich in heart-healthy omega-3 fatty acids and other important vitamins and minerals.

Some processed forms of fat in our food (hydrogenated fat) do affect levels of blood cholesterol. Total blood cholesterol contains both low-density lipoproteins (LDL, bad cholesterol), which deposit fat in artery walls, and high-density lipoproteins (HDL, good cholesterol), which remove cholesterol from the blood. When total blood cholesterol becomes too high, and especially the LDL cholesterol, then risk for heart disease increases.

Trans fats come from plant oils that have been hydrogenated or made more solid, like shortening or margarine. **Trans fats not only raise LDL, they actually lower HDL.** Trans fats are the bad guys! Commercially prepared baked goods, snack foods, and processed foods, including fried fast foods, are high in trans fats. So remember to avoid all processed foods that list hydrogenated or partially hydrogenated oils near the beginning of the ingredient list (including regular peanut butter!). Hydrogenated oils and refined polyunsaturated oils increase the risk of not only heart disease, but also cancer, diabetes, liver disease, dementia, and other diseases.

KNOW THY FATS

Most of the fat in our diet comes in three forms: saturated, polyunsaturated, and monounsaturated.

Saturated Fats

The idea that saturated fats and dietary cholesterol are the major food contributors to heart disease is being revisited. Saturated fats are generally solid at room temperature and are highest in red meats like beef, lamb, and pork. The fats in poultry and fish are less saturated and, therefore, softer than that of beef, lamb, and pork. The fats in whole milk, whole milk products, butter, coconuts, and palm kernels are also sources of saturated fats. Saturated fats have been thought to raise total blood cholesterol, and we have been told that they should be eaten sparingly.

The wisdom of limiting natural saturated fats is now being challenged. Recent evaluation of previous studies related to saturated fat in the diet, especially with traditional populations who have little exposure to Western foods, has yielded some interesting findings. Valuable research begun in the 1930s showed the health benefits of saturated fats in the diet and the detrimental effects of processed foods, which were beginning to become popular. These studies and recent research all seem to indicate that the amount of natural saturated fat in the diet does not correlate with increase in blood cholesterol and heart disease, but the amounts of hydrogenated fats and refined poly-unsaturated oils do. The fact that natural saturated fats in the American diet have decreased by 20% while hydrogenated fats and refined polyunsaturated oils have increased 400% over the same period that obesity, heart disease, and cancer have risen to become the nation's greatest health crises does not seem like a coincidence.

The nutritional benefits of cream and butterfat from grass-fed cows merit special consideration. The fat-soluble vitamins A, D, E, and K are important nutrients that are better absorbed from animal sources. Vitamin A from animal fat is necessary for beta-carotene from plant sources to be converted to vitamin A in our bodies. Natural fat from cream and butter is high in many important fatty acids, but especially omega-3 fatty acids and conjugated linoleic acid (CLA). Research is finding that CLA plays important roles in the immune system, cardiovascular system, nervous system, digestive system, bones and teeth, and lean body mass. Egg yolks from grass-fed chickens have the same nutritional benefits. Grass-fed animals have as much as one-third less total fat than grain-fed animals, but more beneficial fat-soluble vitamins and balance of omega-3 and omega-6 fatty acids!

While the scientists duke it out over saturated fat, we might think again about the culinary delights, if not the potential health benefits, of whole foods like butter, cream, real milk (not homogenized and low pasteurized), real ice cream, and fermented whole milk products (yogurt, kefir, and cheese). We could enjoy eggs, meats, and poultry—and, of all things, cook with tropical oils like palm kernel and coconut! Organic and unrefined natural fats and oils are preferred. Meat and dairy products should preferably be from grass-fed animals, according to God's design—and all in moderation, of course!

Polyunsaturated and Monounsaturated Fats

Polyunsaturated (omega-3 and omega-6) and monounsaturated (omega-9) fatty acids are mostly from plants, fatty fish, and grass-fed animals. They are liquid at room temperature. Omega-3 and omega-6 fatty acids are essential nutrients that cannot be produced by the body in great enough amounts to be beneficial and must be obtained from foods. In the American diet, omega-6 fatty acids are found naturally in vegetables, grains, and legumes, as well as meat, poultry, and eggs. Omega-6 fatty acids have predominated in our diets from overuse of refined oils made from corn, sunflower, safflower, soybean, and cottonseed in the last 30 years. The consumption of farm-raised, grain-fed meats has also increased our intake of omega-6. Omega-3 polyunsaturated fatty acids are found in fish oils, nuts, and seeds—especially walnuts and flax, legumes, olive oil, winter squash, and the fat of grass-fed animals.

The essential polyunsaturated fatty acids omega-6 and omega-3 should be in a ratio of 1 to 1. In the American diet, in which most of our sources of omega-6 fatty acids come from refined oils, the ratio is almost 20:1. Low levels of omega-3 fatty acids and excessive levels of omega-6 fatty acids have been linked to mood disorders (depression, for example), asthma, heart disease, sudden infant death syndrome, and type 2 diabetes. Remember, the best sources of omega-3 polyunsaturated acids are fatty fish or fish oils, flaxseed and walnuts (including their oil), legumes, olive oil, winter squash, and fats from grass-fed animals. The American Heart Association recommends that we eat fatty fish (mackerel, lake trout, herring, sardines, light tuna, and salmon) twice a week. Do not eat albacore or white tuna, shark, swordfish, king mackerel, or tilefish because they contain high levels of mercury.

Americans get plenty of omega-6 polyunsaturated fats from the natural foods that contain them, such as meat, poultry, and eggs. Fat from grass-fed animals, including that in whole milk, cream, butterfat, and egg yolks, is an excellent source of omega-3 fatty acids. These fats also have more of the vitamins

A, D, and E and other natural fatty acids. Refined oils from corn, soy, safflower, and sunflower should be used sparingly because of the high amounts of omega-6 fatty acids they contain and their susceptibility to oxidation.

Monounsaturated fats are found in avocados, almonds, pecans, peanuts, peanut oil, avocado oil, and virgin olive oil. These oils are good—they not only lower LDL, but raise HDL levels and contain a variety of phytochemicals. Extra-virgin, cold-pressed, and unfiltered olive oil will retain the most phytochemicals.

OLIVE OIL

Olive oil is one of the world's healthiest foods! It is, of course, one of the oldest too. Cultivation of olives began about 5000 B.C. Olive oil has been used through the ages for anointing of kings, cosmetics, ointments, medicine, and of course, food. In Genesis 8:11, a dove brought an olive branch to Noah after the flood. This was a symbol that the waters of the flood were receding and that life was returning to earth. In biblical times, olive oil was very important for everyday life, and it was also a part of temple ritual and worship. When God commanded that a tent for meeting with Him be made by the Israelites in the desert, olive oil was specified as the oil to use for the lighting of the eternal lamps (Exodus 27:20). The children of Israel were promised a land where they would acquire, among other things, olive trees that they did not plant (Deuteronomy 6:11).

Modern medicine now knows that virgin olive oil (not refined) has a long list of health benefits. In addition to protecting against heart disease, the nutritional factors in olive oil protect against other chronic degenerative diseases, such as arthritis, cancer, diabetes, and asthma. Olive oil has also been shown to lower blood pressure and help prevent bone loss. Today most commercial olive oil production is still centered in the Mediterranean countries like Spain, Italy, Portugal, Greece, and Turkey. Most all of the olive oil production in the US is in California.

Virgin olive oils should be purchased in dark-tinted bottles only. Choose a bottle toward the back of the shelf. Store olive oil in a cool, dark place (probably the refrigerator). Both light and heat destroy the taste and nutritional value of olive oil. Purchase only as much oil as will be used in three to four months. To protect the olive oil's flavor and nutritional value and to lessen the oxidation that occurs when the oil is exposed to air, transfer to a smaller bottle the amount to be used in the next week or so. Leave this small bottle at room temperature for easy use, but refrigerate the rest. When chilled, olive oil will solidify slightly and turn cloudy, but once restored to room temperature, it will regain its normal appearance, and its quality will have been better maintained.

NUTS AND SUCH

Don't forget that all kinds of nuts and seeds, such as pecans, almonds, walnuts, hazelnuts, macadamia nuts, pistachios, peanuts, sunflower seeds, sesame seeds, pumpkin seeds, and flaxseeds, contain unsaturated plant oils that can add not only health benefits but also variety to our meals and snacks. Nuts and seeds contain not only heart healthy oils but also protein and dietary fiber that give us a feeling of satiety after eating only a small amount. Using nuts and seeds as a snack, combined with other whole foods, such as fruits and vegetables, helps regulate blood sugar levels and helps control hunger. Choose natural (not hydrogenated) nut butters, like old-fashioned peanut butter. Yes, the oil rises to the top, but just stir it up. It's better for us.

Check food labels to be sure the nuts and seeds have not been "roasted" in hydrogenated or partially hydrogenated fat. Try roasting your own. **Remember, the more natural the food, the more nutrients will be available.** Be sure to check serving sizes for nuts and seeds.

Also, food labels can help us choose more unsaturated oils. All food labels by law have to list the amount of trans fat, just as they list total fat, saturated fat, polyunsaturated fat, and monounsaturated fat. Unfortunately, most of the trans fats in the American diet come from fried and fabricated processed foods. That, of course, includes processed crackers, cookies, pastries, cakes, and fried foods at the grocery store or fast-food restaurant. In fact, most fast food and snack food have trans fats. Although natural cholesterol in food does not increase risk for heart disease, cholesterol that has been damaged due to high-temperature processing, such as meats and fats cooked by high-temperature frying, do increase the risk. Powdered milk and eggs, which are added to many processed foods, also contain damaged cholesterol.

REMEMBER!

To substitute healthy fats for unhealthy ones, try these tips:

- Use olive oil instead of polyunsaturated oils for sautés or panfrying.
- Try avocado, sesame, or virgin coconut oil for panfrying.
- Use sesame or peanut oil for quick stir-fry.
- Use a little coconut oil combined with peanut, avocado, sesame, or olive oil for stability when panfrying for any length of time.
- Add walnut or flax oil to salads or marinades.
- Use extra-virgin, cold-pressed, unfiltered olive oil in salad dressings or marinades.
- Use light olive oil (with no taste) for baking.
- Dip bread in extra-virgin, cold-pressed, unfiltered olive oil.
- Use organic butter instead of margarine for spreads.
- Eat fatty fish at least twice a week.
- Add nuts (especially walnuts, peanuts, pecans, and hazelnuts) and seeds (especially flax, pumpkin, and sunflower) to salads, stir-fry, yogurt, cereals (hot or cold), or fruit. Try roasting raw nuts in the oven.
- Use natural nut butters.

- Use organic milk yogurt, kefir, and cheeses.
- Add organic butter and cream to casseroles, sauces, and soups.
- Use organic butter instead of margarine or shortening in baked products.
- Choose organic free-range eggs (eggs from grass-fed poultry).
- Avoid fried processed foods (fast foods or packaged).
- Eat healthy olives, avocados, nuts, and nut butters.

Remember: Use only natural, unrefined fats and oils—no trans fats and no refined polyunsaturated oils.

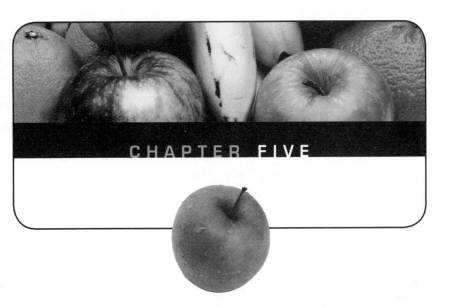

CHAPTER FIVE

PROTEIN: IT'S WHAT'S FOR DINNER

---●---

I will provide grass in the fields for your cattle, and you will eat and be satisfied.
—Deuteronomy 11:15

*"Which of you fathers, if your son asks for a fish, will give him a snake instead?
Or if he asks for an egg, will give him a scorpion?"*
—Luke 11:11–12

PROTEINS are literally the building blocks of our bodies. Every body cell contains protein. Protein forms most body structures, such as skin, nails, hair, membranes, muscles, teeth, bones, organs, ligaments, and tendons. Protein is necessary for growth and tissue repair.

All enzymes and most hormones contain protein. Protein is necessary for the function of the immune system. Protein regulates fluid and acid/base balance. Protein transports nutrients into and out of cells. Protein may also be used by the body for glucose and energy if there is not enough carbohydrate and fat in the diet. Carbohydrate and then fat are the preferred sources of energy. The "protein sparing" function of these energy nutrients saves protein for other more important uses.

Proteins are composed of one or more chains of amino acids. Our bodies use only 20 different amino acids, which are put together in different configurations to make up the thousands of different kinds of proteins we need. Eleven of these amino acids can be manufactured by a healthy body; however, nine of these essential amino acids *must* come from the foods we eat—from good protein sources!

SOURCES OF PROTEIN

Good protein from food comes from both animal and plant sources. Animal sources like dairy products, fish, poultry, eggs, and red meats contain all the amino acids that the body needs to make new proteins. These are called *complete proteins*. Plant sources lack one or more amino acids and are *incomplete proteins*; that means that any plant source of protein, such as legumes, grains, nuts, and seeds, must be combined with something else to make a complete protein. In general, legumes (beans, peas, and lentils) combined with grains, nuts, and seeds make a complete protein. Examples of combinations that provide a complete protein include beans and brown rice, black-eyed peas and stone-ground corn bread, peanut butter and whole wheat bread, hummus and whole wheat pita bread, chili and sesame seed crackers, bean burrito or taco, and lentil and bulgur soup—and there are many more possibilities. Vegans, or strict vegetarians who eat no animal products at all, must combine plant proteins in this manner. Any plant protein can be made complete with the addition of a small amount of complete protein like milk, milk powder, cheese, eggs, and, of course, fish, poultry, or red meat. Millions of Americans today are vegetarians. That's another story altogether! We will look at various aspects of vegetarianism further along this chapter.

Using plant protein sources alone or in combination with meat is also a great way to stretch our budget for meat—usually the most expensive item on our shopping lists! Animal sources of protein can actually be the "garnish" of a recipe, not the main ingredient, and still provide complete protein. Just a small amount of protein in any meal or snack helps give the eater a feeling of fullness and satiety.

As we have seen with other food sources in the United States, time-honored traditions have gone by the wayside for the sake of convenience and the bottom line. In this country, animals raised for meat consumption, including cattle, sheep and lambs, pigs, goats, and chicken, are now not fed as nature intended. Many are in confinement all their lives and are mass-produced, as is most everything else nowadays. These "factory farms" do help lower meat costs, but at a much greater price than we should pay healthwise. Animals raised in confined conditions are given diets designed to boost their productivity and lower costs. The main ingredient is grain, which is kept at artificially low prices by the government. To further cut costs, the feed may contain by-product feed, such as municipal garbage, cookies, poultry manure, chicken feathers, bubble gum, candy bars, and restaurant waste. Until 1997, cattle were also being fed meat that had been trimmed from other cattle—in effect, turning herbivores into carnivores. This unnatural practice is believed to be the underlying cause of mad cow disease.

A high-grain diet can cause physical problems for ruminant animals—cud-chewing animals, such as cattle, dairy cows, goats, and sheep. Ruminants are designed to eat fibrous grasses, plants, and shrubs—not starchy, low-fiber grain. When cattle are switched from pasture to grain, they can become afflicted with a number of disorders, including a common but painful gastrointestinal condition that causes them to kick at their bellies, go off their feed, and eat dirt. To prevent more serious and sometimes fatal reactions, these animals are given chemical additives along with a constant, low-level dose of antibiotics. Some of these antibiotics are the same ones used in human medicine. When medications are overused in the feedlots, bacteria become resistant to them.

Switching ruminants from their natural diet of grasses to grains also lowers the nutritional value of their meat. Grain-fed animals have more total fat, but fewer fat-soluble vitamins and beneficial fatty acids in the fat they have—in other words, more calories and fewer nutrients—as a result of our modern advances in animal technology. Chickens, turkeys, and pigs are also being raised in confinement. Typically, they suffer an even worse fate than ruminants. Tightly packed into cages, sheds, or pens, they cannot practice their normal behaviors, such as rooting, grazing, and roosting. Worse yet, they cannot escape their own manure. Meat and eggs from these animals are also lower in a number of key vitamins and omega-3 fatty acids. On large factory farms where animals are raised in feedlots, the surrounding soil is overloaded with nutrients, resulting in ground and water pollution that causes the "dead zones" in many US coastal areas, as discussed previously.

Supporting local grass-fed meat and egg farms will not only help raise the nutritional value of our food, but also benefit the environment and, by the more humane treatment provided on such farms, the animals. Larger poultry, egg, and meat producers are beginning to feel the pressure to make their products healthier by feeding sources of omega-3 fatty acids to their animals and leaving off the antibiotics and hormones. These products may not be considered completely organic unless they have the USDA Organic seal. However, with the support of consumers, this is a step in the right direction. Many countries, especially in Europe, are way ahead of the United States in demanding natural organic grass-fed meat and dairy products. Hopefully, the US will catch up soon!

CLEAN AND UNCLEAN FOODS

The topic of healthy and unhealthy meats leads us to the discussion of a long-term controversy in the Christian church regarding clean and unclean meats. We won't belabor the point, but beginning with Peter's encounter with the Gentile believers in Acts 10, the question of whether God's food regulations for the Israelites are required of the Christian is still being debated in some circles today. As you may recall, after Noah and his family came out of the ark, God told Noah that just as all plants had been given for food before the flood, after the flood, animals could also be eaten—but not their blood (Genesis 9:3–4). God gave the Israelites a list of animals that were clean or unclean for sacrifice and food in Leviticus 11 and Deuteronomy 14, but God did not say that the list was given for health reasons. He just told the Israelites not to eat the unclean animals, and that was enough—just because He said so! We are not really told why some animals were designated as clean and some unclean. Why would a catfish or shrimp be called unclean and not a carp, since they are all scavengers? Based on today's scientific knowledge, we can't make a case that God restricted the Israelites only from eating harmful meats.

In Leviticus 11:44–45, God does say that since He is holy, He wants his people to be holy and separate—set apart from other cultures. The distinctions of what the Jewish people were to do and not to do regarding cleanliness (food or otherwise) were to remind them of holiness and who they were as a people of God. The Jewish people had rules about what was clean and what was not clean. No other people or nation did. Those rules separated the nation of Israel from Gentile nations.

Jesus and the disciples were certainly practicing Jews and obeyed the food laws. However, as Christianity began to spread to the Gentiles, some major issues had to be resolved about just how Jewish these new Christians were to be! For a fascinating story about how the Jewish Christians abbreviated the food requirements of the Law for the new believers who were Gentiles, read Acts 15.

For a person who desires to follow Christ, the real issue is one of love. Love seeks to build up, never to tear down or to destroy. *"If your brother is distressed because of what you eat, you are no longer acting in love. Do not by your eating destroy your brother for whom Christ died"* (Romans 14:15). We are not to be preoccupied with our Christian liberties, but rather with love. Love never causes a brother to stumble, but seeks to strengthen the weak. Today there are Christians who abstain from eating meats that were considered unclean in the Old Testament. If that is their conviction, then it should be respected. However, brothers who abstain from eating certain meats should not condemn those who do eat those meats.

VEGETARIANISM

This leads us to the discussion of not eating meats at all—in other words, vegetarianism. This was a hot issue in the early church and is still debated and widely practiced today. The same principles of Christian liberty apply here. Whether we agree with the practice of vegetarianism or not, within its realm are several issues related to healthy eating that warrant a look.

In 1997, the American Dietetic Association issued a position statement about vegetarianism: "It is the position of The American Dietetic Association (ADA) that appropriately planned vegetarian diets are healthful, are nutritionally adequate, and provide health benefits in the prevention and treatment of certain diseases."

Vegetarianism can be practiced in many patterns, including the two major patterns: **lacto-ovo-vegetarian pattern,** which is based on grains, vegetables, fruits, legumes, seeds, nuts, dairy products, and eggs and excludes meat, fish, and poultry; and the **vegan pattern** (total vegetarianism), in which all animal products are excluded from the diet. Even within these patterns, considerable variation may exist in the extent to which animal products are avoided. Of course, there are also many people who cut back on all meat or just red meat for various reasons, including expense.

As mentioned before, plant sources of protein can be combined to give an adult plenty of complete protein. Pregnant women, children, and teenagers are another story, however. If a lacto-ovo-vegetarian diet is adopted, chances are very good, even for people in any of these groups, that all the nutrients they need can be supplied, including protein. However, for vegans, who get **no** animal sources of protein, several nutrients could be deficient in the diet of persons in any of these three groups. Adequate protein is extremely important for all pregnant women, children, and teenagers, in whom so much growth is taking place.

In addition to protein, nutrients that vegans should be careful to get enough of include vitamin B_{12}, vitamins A and D, calcium, iron, zinc, and omega-3 fatty acids. Although most of these nutrients (except vitamin B_{12}) are available in plants or can be converted to these nutrients in our bodies from plant sources, the vegan diet does not usually provide enough of them to support good health in most adult vegans, much less pregnant women, children, or adolescents.

However, the diets of many children and teenagers today would make a vegan diet look nutritious! When french fries, soft drinks, and cookies are the mainstays of the diet, there's much room for improvement. A pregnant or breast-feeding woman who is a vegan should be under careful supervision from her obstetrician. Vegan parents should also have a pediatrician carefully watch the growth and nutritional status of their children. Several good resources about vegetarian nutrition are available, including the American Dietetic Association Web site: *www.eatright.org*.

LEGGO MY LEGUMES

Some of the best sources of plant protein and other valuable nutrients are the legumes. Legumes (beans, peas, and lentils) have been cultivated all over the world for thousands of years. Legumes were also an important part of American regional cooking until processed foods took over. We just don't have time for those beans to soak anymore! Our parents and grand-parents grew up eating lots of butter beans, pinto beans, navy beans, and black-eyed peas for good reason. Legumes are cheap and very nutritious. Combined with grains, they make a complete protein. Legumes are among the best sources for dietary fiber in our diet, with some beans and peas contributing in a single serving over half of the fiber we need to eat in one day! Legumes are also rich in minerals and B vitamins. My family loves black beans in any fashion. If you don't have time to cook beans from scratch, just use canned beans. They are good by themselves, in soups, in casseroles, or pureed with herbs and spices for dips. Black bean soup right out of the can is a fast and healthy appetizer, lunch, or snack. Just add some cheese and chopped tomatoes.

Many Americans, especially vegetarians, have begun to consume more and more of one particular super legume—soybeans. The sale and consumption of soy-based products have rocketed in the last few years. For one reason, more soy products are available on the market. For another, consumption of whole soy products in many cultures is linked to healthy living. Soy has been consumed in China and Japan for thousands of years. Of course, the preparation was with traditional methods developed over those millennia. Traditional whole soybean products like Japanese edamame and soybean products like tofu, tempeh, natto, miso, and soy sauce are best. Availability of soy products is expanding in the US.

Although there are health questions about using soy exclusively as a protein source and using processed soy products, soy in moderation is a healthy choice since it also has a wealth of other vitamins, minerals, and phytochemicals. In 1999, the FDA approved food label claims for soy protein related to heart health, although these claims are in review. These claims state that 25 grams of soy protein daily included in a low-saturated-fat diet may help lower heart disease risk. Also, the American Academy of Pediatrics continues to recommend the use of soy protein–based infant formula, but *only* for infants who cannot breast-feed or take milk-based formula. Soy formula for infants should be a last resort.

The health effects of soy isoflavones, plant compounds that are structurally similar to human estrogen, are another issue. Opinions in the scientific community are mixed about isoflavones' ability to reduce risk of breast and prostate cancer, osteoporosis, and menopause symptoms. While some studies have shown that isoflavones give protection against breast and prostate cancer and osteoporosis and relieve hot flashes in menopause, other studies are not conclusive. Until the long-term safety of consuming large amounts of isoflavones is documented, consuming soy products with more than 100 milligrams of isoflavones is unwise. This would mean that about two servings of soy products like edamame, tofu, soy milk, miso, tempeh, or natto would give enough soy protein to be beneficial (25 grams), but not enough to be harmful. Tofu and tempeh, both soy products, make great meat alternatives or meat extenders. Nontraditional processed soy products like textured vegetable protein and meat alternatives (soy "meat" crumbles and imitation hamburgers, hot dogs, sausage, chicken patties and nuggets, bacon, and cold cuts) should be eaten in limited quantities. Soy oil should be avoided. Soy is best consumed as a fermented whole bean or whole bean product. Reading food labels of soy foods is a must, since products vary in amounts of protein and isoflavones due to processing. For whole soy recipes, try the Web sites *www.thesoydailyclub.com* and *www.soyfoods.com* and these books:

- *The Whole Soy Cookbook* by Patricia Greenberg and Helen Newton Hartung
- *Cooking Healthy with Soy* by JoAnna M. Lund and Barbara Alpert
- *Quick and Easy Soy and Tofu Recipes* by Polly Grimaldi

ANIMAL PROTEINS
Animal sources of protein offer a variety of choices for health, budget, and taste. Eggs and low-fat milk products are excellent and inexpensive sources of complete protein. Saturated fat and

cholesterol in egg yolks can be eliminated in recipes by using two whites for one whole egg (or use egg substitutes). Of course, without the color, thickening, and emulsifying functions of the yolk, other ingredients in recipes would have to be adjusted. The yolks, for those who eat them, are packed with high-quality protein, iron, B vitamins, and vitamins A, D, E, and K. Egg yolks also contain phytochemicals. Poultry and fish contain less saturated fat and cholesterol than do red meats. Fish (especially fatty fish) and shellfish also contain large amounts of omega-3 fatty acids, which help prevent heart disease. In addition to being a complete protein, lean red meats are rich in iron and zinc. All animal proteins contain B vitamins. In fact, vitamin B_{12} comes only from animal sources. Lean red meats in moderation are a part of healthy eating. If you have elevated blood lipids (cholesterol, triglycerides), be sure to check with your doctor or registered dietitian about dietary recommendations.

In general, the dietary reference intake (DRI) for protein is 46 grams for women and 56 grams for men daily. Most Americans get at least 70 grams or more per day. Excessive amounts of protein have been linked to heart disease, gout, kidney disease, certain cancers, and calcium loss. One should not consume more than twice the daily DRI for protein on a regular basis. For building muscle in strength training, eating a serving of protein along with carbohydrate from 30 to 45 minutes after a workout can help build and repair muscle. The carbohydrate spares the protein from being burned as energy. Suggestions include a tuna or turkey sandwich, low-fat yogurt, fruit and cottage cheese, egg on toast, cereal and milk, and apple with cheese or peanut butter.

Portion sizes for animal protein are much smaller than we usually think. One portion of lean meat, poultry, or fish is 2 to 3 ounces—about the size of a deck of cards or a tennis ball. A 2-ounce serving of meat provides protein equivalent to ½ cup of beans, 2 eggs, ½ cup of tofu, 2 tablespoons of peanut butter, or 1 ounce of nuts or seeds.

REMEMBER!

Keep in mind these protein facts and recommendations:

- Several kinds of plant proteins combined together provide a complete protein.

- Vegans must be sure to supplement their diet with the essential nutrients they are missing from animal foods.

- No pregnant or lactating mother, child, or teenager should be on a vegan diet.

- Choose organic grass-fed meats and poultry (and eggs of such) when possible; package will indicate **no hormones or antibiotics.**

- Eat fish (especially fatty fish) twice a week.

- Soy infant formula should be used only as last resort.

- Consume no more than two servings of soy products a day.

- Add eggs (especially organic) to dishes as an inexpensive way to add extra protein.

- Animal protein is the **only** source of vitamin B_{12} in the diet.

- For building and repairing muscle mass, eat or drink a serving of protein 30 to 45 minutes after a strength-training workout.

- A single portion of meat, poultry, or fish is only the size of a deck of cards or a tennis ball.

- Supplement or substitute meat with legumes (beans and peas) when possible.

- Use tofu or tempeh as a meat substitute or extender.

- Add nuts and seeds to snacks or dishes to add more protein.

Remember: Protein is essential to health, but a little goes a long way!

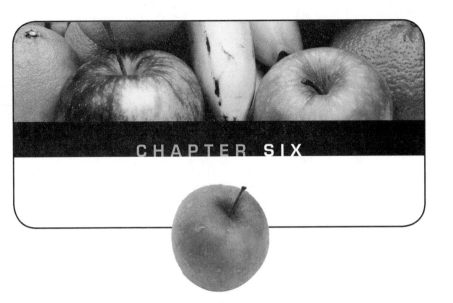

GOT MILK?

●

In that day, a man will keep alive a young cow and two goats.
And because of the abundance of the milk they give, he will have curds to eat.
All who remain in the land will eat curds and honey.
—Isaiah 7:21–22

MILK, curds (yogurt, kefir, and cheese), cream, and butter have been highly valued in cultures around the world for thousands of years. Of course, we are talking about raw fresh milk and its products from grass-fed cows. Pasteurization and homogenization of milk may have changed the nutritional value of all dairy products to some extent, but milk and milk products still remain an important source of valuable nutrients. High-temperature, short-time (HTST) pasteurization, or low pasteurization, preserves more nutrients in the milk than does ultra-pasteurization. Many organic dairies use the HTST process.

Milk and dairy products are one of the major dietary sources of calcium—the most abundant mineral in the body. Calcium is necessary for building and maintaining healthy bones and teeth; it also helps regulate heartbeat, nerve functions, hormone secretions, and clotting of blood. In addition to providing calcium, dairy products are excellent sources of zinc, phosphorus, magnesium, complete protein, B vitamins, and vitamins A and D. Lack of adequate calcium and vitamin D has been associated not only with risk of osteoporosis and osteoarthritis, but also with high blood cholesterol, diabetes, hypertension, multiple sclerosis, autoimmune disease, premenstrual syndrome (PMS), many types of cancer, and obesity. Vitamin A from animal sources, such as milk, butter, cream, and organ meats, is important for vision, growth, bone and teeth development, development and maintenance of skin and mucous membranes, immune function, protection from certain cancers and heart disease, and normal reproduction. Vitamin A is necessary for the metabolism of nutrients in the body, including iron and beta-carotene. In the body, vitamins A and D are absorbed better from whole or low-fat dairy products than from skim.

MILK WITH THE MOST

The trend over the last several generations not to pasture but to grain feed cows has changed the composition of the milk that we drink. In addition to that, the homogenization and ultra-pasteurization of milk over the past 60 years have made what was once a raw, natural, nutritious whole food for many cultures into, well, let's just say a food that is not as whole or nutritious as it once was. Since we are way past the era of one cow per household, we must work within our present culture. Milk and milk products that are HTST pasteurized (not ultra-pasteurized) and not homogenized and come from organic grass-fed cows are about as close as we can come to the kind of dairy products that God intended for us to eat. Studies show that organic pasteurized milk has higher levels of omega-3 fatty acids, 75% higher levels of beta-carotene, and 50% higher levels of vitamin E than does nonorganic milk, and two to three times the level of the antioxidants lutein and zeaxanthin. And even though many farm families in our country still drink raw milk, it is not legal for sale in most states, except for use by animals.

Many artisan farmhouse cheeses are handmade in small batches from HTST pasteurized or raw milk. You might be surprised how many small dairies are located near you. Raw cheese is also readily available online from many sources. However, drinking raw milk or eating raw milk products that are sold commercially is an individual decision, since we really do not "know" that cow! Fermented milk products (yogurt and cheese), which have been around since the beginning (Genesis 18:8), are excellent substitutes that offer the health benefits of raw milk.

Today, common fermented products like buttermilk, yogurt, kefir (similar to drinkable yogurt), and cheeses contain the bacteria we need for gastrointestinal health—bacteria that are killed through pasteurization of raw milk. Yogurt with live cultures and especially kefir are teeming with live friendly bacteria that actually colonize in your gastrointestinal tract. These good bacteria contribute to a healthy immune system, nervous system, and, of course, digestive system. Good bacteria are especially needed during and after the use of antibiotics that kill both good and bad bacteria. Look for active live cultures on the label. You can make your own yogurt and kefir if you want to eliminate the sugars, artificial sweeteners, and additives of commercial products. Some good commercial organic yogurts are made with all-natural ingredients. If no organic dairy product source is located near you, check out the following Web sites:

- www.organicconsumers.org
- www.browncowfarm.com
- www.butterworksfarm.com
- www.stonyfield.com

- *www.heliosnutrition.com*
- *www.lifeway.net*

To maximize the health benefits of yogurt or kefir, eat it plain (no sugar) or mix it with fresh fruit and/or a little jelly or jam. Also, plain natural yogurt or kefir may be mixed with commercial brands to dilute the sugar and other additives in the commercial brands.

GOTTA GET YOUR CALCIUM

Osteoporosis is the most common disease related to the body's need for calcium and vitamin D, and it affects millions of women and some men. Osteoporosis is characterized by thinning of bone tissue. One of every two women is at risk for developing bone fractures after menopause due to osteoporosis; those who are fair-skinned and blond, petite and small boned, underweight or have experienced anorexia nervosa, lactose intolerant, or sedentary are especially at risk. Smoking, alcohol use, and caffeine intake increase osteoporosis risk.

Calcium and vitamin D intake, estrogen replacement therapy, and weight-bearing exercise may all help slow loss of bone as women enter menopause, but the best way to prevent osteoporosis is to eat plenty of calcium-rich foods, beginning in childhood and continuing throughout life. The more calcium put into bones, the more there is to draw from. Calcium is continuously being taken out of skeletal tissues for different bodily functions and must be replaced daily from foods. Research has shown that in the approximate age range of 11 to 16 years, more calcium is stored than at any other time. Even when peak bone mass occurs around the age of 30, it is important to consume adequate calcium to maintain bone mass until menopause or about 50, when more calcium begins to be taken out of bones than can be put back in. After age 50, calcium is needed to help reduce bone loss and prevent osteoporosis.

Calcium from foods must be absorbed by the body with the help of vitamin D. Vitamin D in the diet of many Americans may be lower that previously thought. Consumption of whole dairy products, organ meats, and egg yolks has declined in recent years. Because we avoid sunlight to prevent skin damage and cancer, the sun, one of our natural sources of vitamin D, doesn't benefit us as it might. Africans and other dark-skinned people, the elderly or homebound, people living in northern latitudes, and women who wear extensive coverings are at increased risk. Although fat-free dairy products are fortified with vitamin D, most Americans simply do not get enough.

Because vitamin D deficiency can increase risk of osteoporosis, several kinds of cancer, and other disorders, the recommended intakes of vitamin D are being reviewed. Some studies have shown that moderate sun exposure (without getting sunburned, of course) may be more of a benefit than a risk because it increases levels of vitamin D. Lack of sufficient sunlight for the skin to pro-duce vitamin D from cholesterol made in the liver may also be one cause of high blood cholesterol in some people.

The American Academy of Dermatology suggests that, regard-less of skin type, a broad-spectrum sunscreen (protects against UVA and UVB rays) with a sun protection factor (SPF) of at least 15 should be used year-round. Sunscreens should be used every day if you are going to be in the sun for more than 20 minutes. However, in order to get enough sunlight to produce adequate vitamin D, some studies suggest that an average of 15 minutes a day without sunscreen in the noonday sun is all that most people need. *Then* put sunscreen back on! Increased fortification of foods with vitamin D may also be recommended. In the meantime, if you are at risk or suffer from osteoporosis, diabetes, arthritis, infertility, depres-sion, autoimmune disorders, diabetes, or breast, prostate, colon, or skin cancers, you may want to request a laboratory examination to determine your vitamin D level.

Inadequate intake of calcium is usually the result of eating too few servings of dairy products or low intake of other sources of calcium like homemade broth, greens, canned fish with bones (salmon or sardines), or legumes. The Dietary Reference Intakes from the National Academy of Sciences recommends anywhere from 1,000 to 1,300 milligrams of calcium a day for adolescents and adults depending on age and sex. Most people can get adequate calcium from three to four servings a day of low-fat dairy products and calcium-fortified foods. Postmenopausal women not on hormone replacement therapy would need to eat one more serving a day. One serving of milk or buttermilk (an 8-ounce glass) has 300 milligrams of calcium. You can count these foods as equivalent: 1 cup of yogurt, 2 ounces of most cheeses, 3 ounces of canned sardines or pink salmon with bones, 1 cup of tofu, and 8 ounces of calcium-fortified orange juice. Dark green leafy vegetables, broth from bones (chicken, meat, or fish), dried fruits like figs, dried beans, nuts, and seeds also contain good amounts of calcium. Homemade broth or stock from chicken or other meat with bones is a rich source of calcium from the bone marrow. To learn to make homemade broth or stock, ask your grandmother or consult a classic reference like *The Fannie Farmer Cookbook* by Marion Cunningham. That generation knew a bunch about broth and stocks! Also, check out *A Great Bowl of Soup* by Christine Byrnes; this new cookbook gives the basics plus additional soup ideas. Whole foods that are rich in calcium are usually also good sources of magnesium and phosphorus, which are important minerals related to bone health and osteoporosis.

EAT DAIRY PRODUCTS, LOSE WEIGHT

One of the most exciting areas of calcium research is that of weight management. A body of evidence is building that suggests that at least 1,000 milligrams of calcium from milk and dairy products combined with a reduced-calorie diet can result in a reduction of body fat in children and adults. Dairy foods seem to produce much more of a loss in weight and body fat than supplementary sources of calcium. The antiobesity effect of dietary calcium has been shown in cellular research as well as animal studies, human epidemiological studies, and clinical trials.

One unexpected finding in some studies has been that more than 50% of total fat lost was from the abdominal region. The central obesity (apple shape) common in men and postmenopausal women is a risk factor for metabolic syndrome, which includes heart disease, hypertension, insulin resistance (a precursor for type 2 diabetes), and type 2 diabetes. Research has shown that exercise and a meal pattern low in refined carbohydrates can drastically reduce the risk from these diseases. We now know that the addition of low-fat dairy products can increase loss of not only total body fat, but abdominal fat. The difference in reduction of body fat with dairy products as opposed to calcium supplements or products fortified with calcium seems to be other components in dairy products besides calcium that work synergistically with the calcium to accelerate burning of fat. The same benefits can be found in organic low-pasteurized whole milk and milk products. Remember that the fatty acids of animals that are grass-fed contain conjugated linoleic acid (CLA), which promotes building of lean body mass instead of fat deposition.

The National Institute of Child Health and Human Development (NICHD) refers to osteoporosis as a "pediatric disease with adult consequences." Only about 10% to 25% of children and adolescents are meeting their calcium requirements. Replacement of milk and dairy products by sweetened beverages lowers the intake in children and adolescents of calcium and other essential nutrients found in a nutrient-dense diet. Intake of high-calorie/low-nutrient-dense foods like sugared beverages leads to obesity but malnourishment in children and adolescents, as well as adults. Children need the extra nutrients from whole milk, and so do growing adolescents. However, in the teen years, low-fat dairy products may be used more and more if desired. The important issue is replacing empty calories from sugared beverages with nutritious dairy foods.

EXERCISE FOR STRONGER BONES

One of the most important factors related to bone health at any age is weight-bearing exercise and strength training. Research suggests that exercise in children and adolescents during bone-forming years helps build bones that are stronger and denser. In fact, some studies have shown that prepubescent children who exercised regularly developed bones that were twice as dense as those in children who did not. Exercise throughout life promotes bone health and slows bone loss even after menopause.

LACTOSE INTOLERANCE

From 30 to 50 million Americans are lactose intolerant according to the American Dietetic Association. This means that they cannot digest the carbohydrate in milk called lactose. Individuals experience varying degrees of intolerance to lactose and thus may have a range of symptoms after eating dairy products. Eating fermented dairy products and cheese may be better tolerated than drinking milk. Products that include the enzyme lactase are also available for dealing with lactose intolerance. Lactose intolerance is easily managed, especially with the help of a registered dietitian.

Calcium and vitamin D supplementation may be necessary for persons with lactose intolerance and for others who do not eat enough dairy products (three to four servings) daily to meet calcium requirements. Pregnant women, adolescents, and the elderly may fit into this category. Calcium supplements in a wide variety are available over the counter. Here are some tips in choosing the one that is best for you:

- Choose known brand names that have the United States Pharmacopeia (USP) symbol.
- Avoid calcium from unpurified products without the USP symbol.
- To test absorption, place a tablet in a small amount of warm water for 30 minutes. If it doesn't dissolve, it will probably not dissolve in the stomach.
- Chewable and liquid supplements dissolve well.
- Calcium is best absorbed by the body if taken several times a day in amounts of 500 milligrams at a time.

- Calcium carbonate is best absorbed when taken with food.
- Calcium citrate can be taken anytime.
- Calcium supplements can cause gas or constipation, so increase supplements slowly.
- Ask your physician if the calcium supplement you choose can cause an interaction with your other medications.

Organic milk and dairy products used to make healthy snacks and desserts can help increase calcium intake in all ages. Add yogurt, cream, or crème fraîche to fresh fruit, or make custards or puddings for delicious, nutrient-dense ways to nourish your body naturally. Make your own crème fraîche by mixing 1 cup of whipping cream with 2 tablespoons of buttermilk. Pour this mixture into a glass jar and cover. The cream will have to stand at room temperature (about 70°F) for 8 to 24 hours until thickened. Crème fraîche can then be refrigerated. It will last about ten days.

REMEMBER!

Dairy products contribute to good health.

- Enjoy at least three servings (three 8-ounce cups) of dairy products each day.
- Children need organic whole dairy products.
- Adolescents and adults may choose from low-fat dairy products.
- Consume organic low-pasteurized, nonhomogenized milk when possible.
- Increase the intake of fermented organic dairy products, such as buttermilk, yogurt, kefir, and cheese, when possible.
- For adequate vitamin D production, which is necessary for calcium absorption and metabolism, spend some time (approximately 15 minutes) in the sun every day with hands and face exposed.

Remember: Eat three servings of dairy products each day.

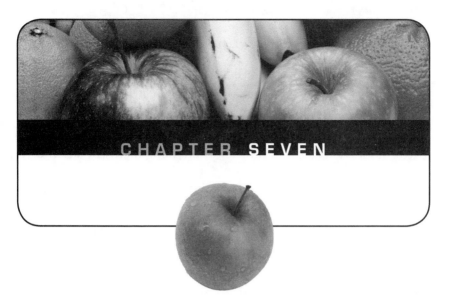

CHAPTER SEVEN

EAT THE LOCAL RAINBOW

●

*When they reached the Valley of Eshcol, they cut off a branch bearing
a single cluster of grapes. Two of them carried it on a pole between them,
along with some pomegranates and figs.*
—Numbers 13:23

*They found an Egyptian in a field and brought him to David.
They gave him water to drink and food to eat—part of a cake of pressed figs
and two cakes of raisins. He ate and was revived.*
—1 Samuel 30:11–12

EAT your fruits and vegetables—these very words
have resounded through many generations...and not
just from the mothers! The story of Daniel and other
young Israelite men who were in captivity with him in

Babylon is told in Daniel 1:1–15. When he and his friends were provided the rich food from the king's table, Daniel asked the chief court official for permission not to eat it but to be given only vegetables and water instead. A ten-day test was permitted. At the end, Daniel and his friends appeared healthier and better nourished than any of the other young men who ate the king's food.

Since the discovery of vitamins 200 years ago, scientists continue to find compounds in fruits and vegetables that protect against disease. Fruits and vegetables are rich sources of dietary fiber, vitamins and minerals (especially antioxidants), and phytochemicals; this makes whole fresh fruits and vegetables powerful deterrents against heart disease, stroke, high blood pressure, and certain cancers.

Scientists have discovered that thousands of plant pigments color foods and that the more colorful they are, the more powerful effect they have on health. Color pigments are categorized into five groups of colors: blue/purple, green, white, yellow/orange, and red.

Blue and purple pigments are rich sources of the phytochemicals anthocyanins and ellagic acids. These phytochemicals work like antioxidants to protect against heart disease, loss of memory function, and certain cancers. Blueberries, purple cabbage, purple grapes, raisins, eggplant, and purple peppers have these pigments.

Green-pigmented produce contains chlorophyll, which masks other colors containing powerful phytochemicals like beta-carotene, lutein, indoles, and sulphoraphane. These pigments protect against cancers, heart disease, stroke, blindness, and lung disease. Some examples are green leafy vegetables, avocados, kiwifruit, asparagus, broccoli, green cabbages, green peppers, green peas, okra, and fresh herbs.

White pigments contain the phytochemicals allium compounds and indoles. Fruits and vegetables that contain white pigments include bananas, white peaches, cauliflower, garlic, ginger, onions, mushrooms, turnips, and white corn. These foods reduce risks of developing certain cancers, heart disease, and stroke.

Yellow and orange pigments include antioxidants like vitamin C and phytochemicals like beta-carotene, hesperidin, tangeritin, and limonene. These pigments help maintain heart health, vision, and the immune system and lower risk of certain cancers. All citrus fruits, yellow apples, apricots, mangoes, papayas, peaches, pineapples, winter and summer squash, carrots, yellow peppers, sweet potatoes, and yellow tomatoes are rich sources.

Powerful red pigments contain lycopene, resveratrol, anthocyanins, quercetins, and ellagic acid that protect heart and urinary tract health and memory function, as well as lower risk of certain cancers. Fruits and vegetables containing these pigments include red apples, cherries, cranberries, red grapes, red pears, raspberries, strawberries, watermelon, beets, red peppers, radishes, radicchio, red onions, rhubarb, and tomatoes.

Try this beet treat: Sauté one or two grated raw beets in a little butter until tender. Add 1 tablespoon of vinegar, 3 tablespoons of sugar, and 2 teaspoons of cornstarch dissolved in ¼ cup of water. Season with salt and pepper. Cook until the sauce clears. Even your children will love these powerful beets!

SPICY TIPS

Herbs and spices cover the range of the color spectrum. Most culinary herbs are green and are leaves of low-growing shrubs. Examples are parsley, chives, marjoram, thyme, basil, caraway, dill, oregano, rosemary, savory, sage, and celery leaves. Spices come from the bark (cinnamon), root (ginger, onion, garlic), buds (cloves, saffron), seeds (yellow mustard, poppy, sesame), berry (black pepper), or the fruit (allspice, paprika) of tropical plants and trees.

Seasoning blends are mixtures of spices and dried herbs. Check spice companies for exact mixtures. Here are some well-known seasoning blends:

- Chili powder: red pepper, cumin, oregano, salt, and garlic powder
- Curry powder: coriander, turmeric, cumin, fenugreek seed, white pepper, allspice, yellow mustard, red pepper, and ginger
- Poultry seasoning: white pepper, sage, thyme, marjoram, savory, ginger, allspice, and nutmeg
- Pumpkin pie spice: cinnamon, ginger, nutmeg, allspice, and cloves

Whole dried herbs and spices last much longer than crushed or ground forms. Many consumers prefer to buy the whole form and crush or grind as needed for greater freshness. Dried herbs and spices can be crushed with a mortar and pestle, by using a rolling pin with spices between two cloths, by using the back of a spoon in a cup, or by using a food processor or coffee grinder. Check ground or crushed herbs and spices for freshness at least once a year. If no aroma is detected after crushing, the seasoning needs to be replaced.

Storage practices make a difference in maintaining the quality of dried herbs and spices:

- Store dried herbs and spices away from moisture in tightly covered, airtight containers. Use clean, dry spoons for measuring.
- Store in a cool place away from sunlight or heat sources, such as the cooking areas or the dishwasher. In hot climates, store spices in the refrigerator or freezer to maintain their quality.

The general ratio for substituting fresh herbs for dried is three to one. In other words, use three times more of a fresh herb than the recipe calls for of a dry herb. To preserve their flavor, fresh herbs are usually added toward the end in cooked dishes. Add the more delicate herbs—basil, chives, cilantro, dill leaves, parsley, marjoram, and mint—a minute or two before the end of cooking or sprinkle them on the food before it is served. The less delicate herbs—dill seeds, oregano, rosemary, tarragon, and thyme—can be added about the last 20 minutes of cooking. Check out these books about herbs and spices:

- *Herb Mixtures and Spicy Blends* by Deborah Balmuth
- *The Contemporary Encyclopedia of Herbs and Spices: Seasonings for the Global Kitchen* by Tony Hill
- *The Herbal Kitchen: Cooking with Fragrance and Flavor* by Jerry Traunfeld

THE VALUE AND USE OF HERBS

For thousands of years, man has been aware of the benefits of herbs and spices for their nutritional value, for their religious value, and for culinary and medicinal purposes. Thousands of years B.C. the Greeks, Egyptians, Hebrews, and Chinese were already putting their knowledge of herbs on paper. Through the centuries, the lists of useful plants for relieving all sorts of ailments and diseases grew longer and longer. The ceremonial and religious use of herbs and spices is referenced throughout the Bible. God told Moses to make a holy anointing oil of myrrh, cinnamon, cane, cassia, and olive oil that was to be used to anoint the tabernacle, the ark of the testimony and other items in the Holy of Holies, and the priests (Exodus 30:23–30). The 2 Chronicles 16:14 description of the burial of Asa, king of Judah, states, *"They laid him on a bier covered with spices and various blended perfumes."* Myrrh played a role in the birth (Matthew 2:11), death (Mark 15:23), and burial (John 19:39) of Jesus. In Matthew, Mark, and Luke, we see that Jesus mentioned common garden herbs in His teachings. Throughout history, herbs and spices have brought extra richness to life.

Today, many Americans are rediscovering the value of fresh herbs in everyday cooking, as so many have done throughout the ages. We may not all have a vegetable garden, but we can all have an herb garden—all you need is a window box! Remove the herbs from their containers, and place them in the window box about four inches apart. Fill in around them with potting soil. Plants will need to be watered at least once a day and regularly fertilized with an organic fertilizer high in nitrogen. The best place for an herb window box is in a sunny area, ideally within easy reach of the kitchen. Possibilities for window-box herbs include basil, chervil, chives, coriander, mint, parsley, rosemary, sage, thyme, tarragon, bay leaves, marjoram, and oregano.

Of course, herbs may also be grown in containers on a patio, balcony, or terrace. Container plants are easily transported and can be arranged in attractive groupings with containers of flowering plants. Herbs in containers also need watering every day. On hot sunny days, they need a second shower. During the growing season, pinch the plants back to keep them bushy and compact, and remove any dead or diseased leaves to keep them healthy.

If you are a gardener, you may already have an herb garden. If not, consider planting one. Herbs are a beautiful and healthy addition to your flowering plants.

Fresh herbs are now usually available at most grocery stores and farmers markets for persons without the time or patience to grow their own.

KEEP NUTRIENTS, AVOID PESTICIDES—BUY LOCAL

The growing conditions, selection, preparation, and storage of fruits and vegetables greatly affect the nutrient content available in our food. The closer the consumer is to the place where the produce is grown and harvested, the more nutrient value is available. That means that locally grown produce is best. Some nutrients are compromised in holding and shipping of produce. It is *best* to eat produce in season, but for fruits and vegetables that are not grown locally, there is no choice. However, enough out-of-season produce is available within the US that there is really no reason to buy imported fruits and vegetables.

Food safety is another concern. Produce grown outside the US may contain more pesticide residue than that grown in the US. In general, fresh strawberries, raspberries, cherries, apples, peaches, nectarines, grapes, spinach, and peas tend to be most contaminated by pesticides. Washing with clean drinking water removes most bacteria and pesticide residue. Also take off outer leaves of vegetables. But the very best way to avoid pesticides is to buy organic produce. Organic foods must—by law—be grown without the use of chemical pesticides and fertilizers. Going organic has become much more popular in the last few years, and organic foods have become more available in the marketplace. Most large supermarket chains now have organic food sections, including organic produce sections, in their stores. Even organic produce must be washed to remove dirt and other bacterial sources. And it is a good idea to *rewash* bagged greens! Washed greens are dried most effectively with a salad spinner.

In the long run, buying locally grown produce is probably more important than buying organic produce. Look for farmers markets in your community. During the summer when the harvest is bountiful, enjoy family outings to a market! Children and grandchildren have fun choosing, preparing, and eating those fresh fruits and vegetables. Yum! Check out these books for recipes:

- *Local Flavors* by Deborah Madison and Laurie Smith
- *Farmer's Market Cooking* by Sally Ann Berk

NEXT BEST TO FRESH

If fresh produce is not available, choose frozen or canned fruits and vegetables. Frozen produce is flash frozen to preserve as many nutrients as possible. Canned produce is subjected to heat that may destroy some nutrients, but eating canned fruits and vegetables is much better than not eating them at all. In fact, some people prefer the taste and consistency of canned vegetables and fruits, especially if they grew up eating such!

Be sure that frozen packages of produce do not look or feel as though they have been thawed and refrozen. When shopping for frozen vegetables, select packages that are not a solid block and the products inside can be felt to be separate pieces. Follow this same rule at home. If the frozen vegetables have formed a solid lump, throw them out; the solid lump is indication that, at some point, the temperature was low enough for the individual pieces to defrost before refreezing. When frozen properly, vegetables and potatoes can be stored in the freezer for up to eight months.

Before purchasing canned goods and before using them after being stored, inspect them for signs of rust or bulging, and discard immediately if either sign is found. Typically, canned goods can be stored for up to one year.

One of my favorite soups in the fall and winter is pumpkin. You may bake the pumpkin, but a quick and easy recipe combines a 15-ounce can of pureed pumpkin with one onion sautéed in a little butter. Add 3 cups of chicken stock and 1 cup of cream, and season to taste. Then it's ready to eat!

JUICING IT UP

Fruit and vegetable juices should be 100% juice, with no sugar or HFCS added. Better yet, can your own juice. Even fresh fruit juices that are juiced at home contain so much natural sugar that they should be enjoyed in small quantities and with other foods. Some new 100% commercial juices, such as pomegranate juice, are powerhouses of antioxidants and phytochemicals. Check out these juices at *www.pomwonderful.com.*

REMEMBER!

Eat your fruits and vegetables!

- When choosing fresh produce, always look for signs of freshness: heavy for size (denotes moisture) and bright colors with no bruising or wilting. For fruits, the aroma should be an indication of quality.

- Use produce as soon as possible, but most vegetables and fruits can be stored a short time in the refrigerator crisper or moisture-proof bags in the refrigerator. Store potatoes, onions, and garlic in a dry, cool, dark area.

- Wash produce in drinking water without soaking.

- Leave peels intact when possible to retain dietary fiber and nutrients.

- Cut produce only when ready to serve or cook, as oxidation and light destroy many nutrients.

- Cook in the least amount of water possible or microwave, steam, or stir-fry. If cooked in water, use the water in preparation, since the water-soluble nutrients remain in the water.

- Heat destroys nutrients, so the quickest cooking time possible is optimal.

- If fresh produce is not available, frozen or canned fruits and vegetables are fine to use, especially if no salt or sugar has been added.

- Fruit and vegetable juices should be 100% juice, with no sugar or HFCS added. Better yet, can your own juice.

- Even fresh fruit juices should be enjoyed in small quantities and with other foods.

Remember: Count the colors on your plate. Eat five to nine servings of colorful fruits and vegetables each day! In other words, eat the local rainbow!

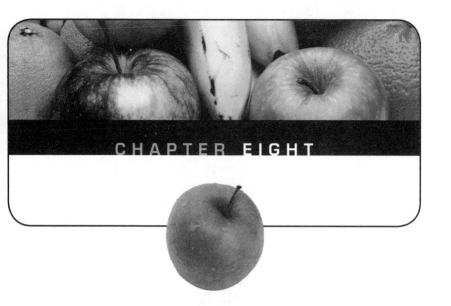

CHAPTER EIGHT

DRINKING TO OUR HEALTH

---•---

"Come, all you who are thirsty, come to the waters; and you who have no money, come, buy and eat! Come, buy wine and milk without money and without cost."
—Isaiah 55:1

IF we are what we eat (and drink), then water is a most important nutrient, even more so than food.

WHY IS WATER SO IMPORTANT?

Next to oxygen, water is the element that is most important to our survival. Our bodies can go for over a month without food, but just a few days without water.

The body weight of a normal adult is 60% to 70% water! Blood is mostly water, and our muscles, lungs, and brain all contain a lot of water. Water is needed to regulate body temperature and to provide the means for nutrients to travel to all our organs. Water also transports oxygen and nutrients to our cells. It removes waste and protects our joints and organs. Water is the medium for the chemical reactions of metabolism in every cell of our body. To fill our need for water, we drink—straight water as well as other beverages. But food is mostly water too—even meat, poultry, and fish. A daily general guide for water intake is about 8 glasses for women and 12 glasses for men—that includes water from other beverages and food intake. When a person is physically active for prolonged periods, especially in high heat and humidity, water loss will increase and the need for water intake will likewise increase.

Usually, if you satisfy your thirst, you will be well hydrated. However, as people age, they may lose their sense of thirst and become dehydrated before feeling thirsty.

Symptoms of mild dehydration include chronic pains in joints and muscles, lower back pain, headaches, and constipation. A strong odor to the urine, along with a yellow or amber color, indicates inadequate water intake.

On the other hand, it is possible to drink too much water. Water intoxication can dilute the body's electrolytes, causing confusion, coma, and death. It may be the cool thing to do, but walking around with your designer water bottle may only send you to the "necessary" more frequently!

The best source of water is plain, pure drinking water. There has been an ongoing debate among scientists about the mineral content of drinking water in the US. For almost 30 years, a group of scientists has been trying to make "hard water," rich in magnesium and calcium, a standard for public water. Even mineral water in the US has low magnesium and calcium. The ideal bottled water should be rich in magnesium and calcium and have low sodium content. Because there is great variation in the mineral content of commercially available bottled waters, the actual mineral content of bottled water should be considered when selecting one for consumption. The best would be natural spring water bottled at the source. European bottled water is typically higher in desired minerals than water bottled in the US. Because of the possibility of high mineral content, mineral water should probably not be given to infants and children. However, for adults, mineral water can be a good source of both magnesium and calcium, both of which tend to be low in American diets.

Local municipal water suppliers can provide information on the hardness level of the water they deliver. If you have a private water supply, you can have the water tested for mineral content. Magnesium levels in municipal drinking waters vary; for instance, they are much higher in Arizona and New Mexico and lower in Florida. Water as a source of magnesium could be valuable, since so many diets lack fruits, vegetables, and whole grains. The increase in consumption of processed foods and phosphates in cola drinks has also substantially reduced magnesium intake.

So what else besides water should we drink for health? We have already discussed why moderation should be used (especially by children) in the consumption of fruit juices because of the high natural sugar content in juices. We also know that not only children but adults also should try to have at least three servings of milk and dairy products daily. Later we will be discussing why soft drinks, whether regular or sugar free, should be limited. So what is left?

TEATIME

Let's talk about tea—afternoon or otherwise. Afternoon tea is a great pick-me-up at about 4:00 P.M., as long as healthy foods are served with it! Actually, next to water, tea is the most-consumed beverage in the world. Research in the past few years has shown that tea leaves have powerful antioxidant and phytochemical properties. Tea also contains caffeine, but much less than coffee. Green tea (unfermented), oolong tea (partially fermented), and black tea (fermented) have many health benefits. Herbal teas, which are derived from different plants, are also beneficial.

Green, oolong, and black tea contain flavonoids and phytochemicals that are, in many cases, the same antioxidants found in fruits and vegetables. In fact, a cup of tea has greater than five times the antioxidant power of most fruits and vegetables. The addition of sweeteners or milk to tea does not seem to lessen the health benefits of a two-cups-a-day tea habit, which can reduce the risk for cancer, heart disease, and stroke.

Herbal teas have been used throughout history for their medicinal benefits. Herbal medicine is the primary form of medicine for perhaps as much as 80% of the world's population. Scientific interest in herbal medicine in the United States has lagged behind that in other countries. In Germany, for example, one-third of graduating physicians have studied herbal medicine, and a comprehensive therapeutic guide to herbal medicines has long been published there. Studies have shown that individual herbal ingredients have specific physical effects, such as calming and relaxing or stimulating and warming, and that certain herbs can benefit specific conditions. Valerian, for example, has been shown to have a relaxing effect and has been used successfully to treat people with anxiety and insomnia. Ginger, which relieves nausea, is now widely used to relieve morning and travel sickness. For all you ever wanted to know about tea, go to *www.twinings.com*. Also, some great books about tea have been published:

- *The New Tea Book: A Guide to Black, Green, Herbal, and Chai Tea* by Sara Perry
- *Herbal Teas: 101 Nourishing Blends for Daily Health and Vitality* by Kathleen Brown and Jeanine Pollak
- *20,000 Secrets of Tea: The Most Effective Ways to Benefit from Nature's Healing Herbs* by Victoria Zak
- *Tea: Discovering, Exploring, Enjoying* by Hattie Ellis

FOR COFFEE LOVERS

Coffee, the "other stimulant," has also been around for thousands of years. The modern-day coffeehouse has become a gathering place. Caffeine, coffee's main ingredient, is a mild, addictive stimulant. Just like cola, coffee has significant amounts of caffeine—about twice that of tea and chocolate. The amount of caffeine in coffee does have modest cardiovascular effects, such as increased heart rate, increased blood pressure, and occasional irregular heartbeat, in some people.

The negative effects of coffee tend to appear with excessive use, so it is best to avoid heavy consumption. However some negative effects occur even without heavy consumption. For some people, even the average dose of caffeine, as found in two cups of coffee, shortens sleep time and increases rapid eye movement sleep (REM sleep). High doses of caffeine can cause nausea, diarrhea, insomnia, trembling, and sensory disturbances. Studies suggest regular caffeine use can contribute to the onset and discomfort of fibrocystic breast disease. Regular coffee drinkers experience physical dependence on caffeine and may suffer withdrawal symptoms, including tension headaches and irritability, which tend to go away in a few days. Many coffee drinkers also have a psychological dependence on caffeine, feeling they need a cup or two in the morning to get going. Caffeine increases dopamine release, which can create dependence as with alcohol, sugar, or exercise. If you feel you could be dependent on caffeine and drink more than four cups of coffee a day, talk with your physician about cutting back. The same approach would apply if you were drinking that many cola beverages a day to keep you going. So with coffee, as with other caffeinated drinks, moderation is the key.

On a positive note, coffee has antioxidants and phytochemicals, as do tea and cocoa. For health benefits, drinking decaffeinated coffee might be best.

DON'T DRINK YOUR CALORIES

Regular colas, which also have caffeine, are a major source of the 100 to 160 pounds of sugar that the average American consumes each year. Other sugared drinks, too, like sweetened fruit juice, punch, or sweet tea, are really nothing but liquid calories. Although liquids may contain calories, they don't seem to satisfy hunger even if they quench the thirst. Physiologically, thirst is quenched once the blood volume and cell volume are increased by water. This sends signals to the brain that a person is no longer thirsty—but it does not change the hunger status. Liquids travel more quickly than food through the intestinal tract; so when drinking a large quantity of beverage, even if it has the same number of calories as a whole regular meal, the satiety signals do not go off. Keep this in mind: a 44-ounce soft drink is 800 calories. Try that on for size!

It's always better to eat the calories than to drink them. Those upscale coffee drinks that sound so inviting and Italian are the equivalent of a hot milk shake. Some contain as many calories (more than 500) as a whole meal, without any of the nutrients. We will be discussing empty calories. Meanwhile, let me tell you: A sweetened beverage is the *poster child* for empty calories! And don't forget sweet tea, Southerners. If it is commercial, it is most likely sweetened with HFCS to the tune of 120 calories for 12 ounces and 33 grams of sugar.

DRINK TO HEALTH

I want to say strongly that **Americans are not drinking healthy beverages**. Statistics show that, on average, Americans drink five times as many sodas and nearly twice as much beer as Europeans. Europeans drink three times as much tea, three times as much wine, and **four times as much tap water** as Americans. So what should we drink? More water, of course. It may be tap water—straight or filtered. Bottled or mineral water is another choice—whether still (no carbonation) or sparkling. When in Venezuela, our family began drinking sparkling water, adding lemon or lime. Now the citrus flavor comes in the water! But I still like the real thing. I like sparkling juices for special occasions or just with Italian food. All **100% fruit juices** are good...in moderation. Tomato juice and fruit and vegetable mixes are great choices. Regular and herbal teas are great for health. Hey, Southerners, I haven't forgotten you. Try sweetening iced tea with stevia, a natural sweetener that is virtually calorie free and is used extensively worldwide; however, be aware that it has not at the time of this book's printing been approved as a sweetener by the US Food and Drug Administration (FDA). If using artificial sweetener or sugar, use it in moderation. If sugar, prepare to walk it off—literally. It's your choice!

REMEMBER!

Drink to your health.

- Next to oxygen, water is the element that is most important to our survival.
- Ideal bottled water is rich in magnesium and calcium and has low sodium content.
- Regular and herbal teas are great for health. A cup of tea has greater than five times the antioxidant power of most fruits and vegetables.
- Avoid drinking empty calories.
- Keep drinking the milk, as well—three servings a day!

Remember: Hydrate when you are thirsty, but don't drink empty calories!

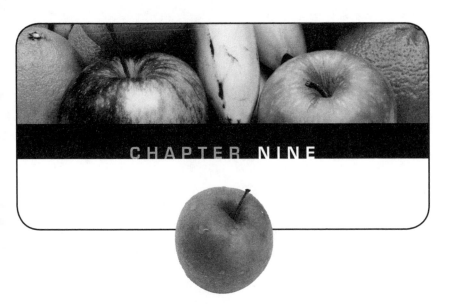

CHAPTER NINE

BREAKFAST OF CHAMPIONS

Jesus said to [the disciples], "Bring some of the fish you have just caught...."
" Come and have breakfast."... Jesus came, took the bread and gave it to them,
and did the same with the fish.
—John 21:10, 12–13

FISH, vegetables, soup, nuts—for breakfast? Yes, and much more! Why? Because the important point is not what *foods* are eaten for breakfast, but what *nutrients* are in those foods. After a night's rest, the body has been without an energy source for 8 to 12 hours. Breakfast is the first chance to refuel and raise those glucose levels that are the brain's and the body's main energy source. Food energy from breakfast begins fueling muscles for the physical activity of the day, helps concentration and problem-solving ability, may help improve memory, and may speed up metabolic rate. In addition, recent research has shown that breakfast eaters are less likely to develop metabolic syndrome (central obesity, hypertension, high blood cholesterol, and insulin resistance).

BREAKFAST FOR CHILDREN

Evidence about the importance of breakfast for children has been building for decades. The School Breakfast Program (SBP), which provides one-fourth or more of a child's daily nutrients, began in 1966 as the relationship between food, good nutrition, and children's ability to develop and learn was recognized.

Studies conclude that students who eat school breakfast show a general increase in math and reading scores as well as improvements in speed and memory in cognitive tests. They perform better on standardized tests than those who skip breakfast **or eat breakfast at home.** They eat more fruits, drink more milk, and consume less saturated fat than those who don't eat breakfast or have breakfast at home. Other studies have shown that children who eat breakfast have higher overall nutrient intakes compared with those who skip breakfast—in other words, the breakfast skippers do not make up for lost nutrients later in the day.

A school breakfast must include milk, a vegetable or fruit or 100% juice from either, two servings of bread or cereal, and a 2-ounce serving of meat or other high-protein food like peanut butter or eggs. High-sugar, low-fiber cereals, tarts, and bars with sugared drinks are common in home breakfasts. Research has shown that a breakfast of refined carbohydrates lasts only one to two hours. A mixed diet combining complex carbohydrate (dietary fiber), protein, and fat provides a feeling of fullness or satiety and the energy needed throughout the morning.

BREAKFAST AND EXERCISE

Breakfast is especially important for those who work out early. A workout before breakfast actually burns more fat, since carbohydrate stores are low after an overnight fast. A light preexercise meal of something like an apple with peanut butter or a cup of yogurt with fresh strawberries provides the carbohydrates the body needs for the workout. Remember that a light postexercise meal of complex carbohydrate and protein helps replenish and build muscles if eaten within about an hour after the workout. Since liquids also need replenishing, this is a good time to include at least a cup or two of milk, milk smoothie, or drinkable yogurt.

CEREALS PLUS

Whole grain products, dairy products, and lean meat proteins or plant proteins provide the energy nutrients needed in breakfast. A perfect example would be the champion of breakfasts in the US—a bowl of whole grain cereal and milk. Remember that not all breakfast cereals are created equal. Label reading is a must for hot or dry cereals. Look for high-fiber cereals that list *100% whole* or *100% whole stone ground* as the descriptor of the first ingredient, which should be a grain like wheat or oats. Bran cereals or those with bran included are also excellent choices. Look for at least 3 grams of dietary fiber per serving, although some have up to 14 grams. Kefir or yogurt combined with cottage or ricotta cheese is also an excellent medium for mixing up dry cereal. Eating oatmeal (not instant or quick) is one of the best ways to start the day. Fruit (for example, apples and/or raisins) and nuts (pecans or walnuts perhaps) may be added to enhance the flavor and increase nutritional value. Slow cookers are a great way to prepare hot breakfast cereals; let them cook overnight, and they are ready to eat the next morning. For some great recipes that cook while you sleep, do a Web search for *slow cooker oatmeal*.

BROADEN THE DEFINITION OF *BREAKFAST FOOD*

Breakfast means many things in other cultures. Americans should consider examples of breakfast foods from other countries and incorporate them into their traditional breakfast routine. In Eastern Europe, Asia, Greece, Turkey, and Africa, soups and porridges that contain meat, poultry, fish, or soy plus vegetables, beans, rice, or noodles may comprise breakfasts. In the Middle East, Greece, and Turkey, yogurt, goat cheese, vegetables (sometimes a salad), nuts, and seeds may be eaten at breakfast. In Northern Europe and Canada, cheeses, cold meats, sausages, vegetables, boiled eggs, and hot cereals are common. In addition, in most countries, various fruits and bread products are usually eaten, and variations of coffee and tea are consumed.

Adding some nontraditional foods to the usual American breakfast choices might be nutritious and delicious! Almost any kind of soup or stew that is usually eaten at another meal is appropriate for breakfast. In fact, leftovers of all kinds are quick and nutritious choices—meat, chicken, fish, vegetables, brown rice, or pasta from durum wheat (semolina). They can be eaten as is or combined with eggs in different ways. Cheese, turkey products, or soy products may also be added. Leftover thin-crust pizza or casserole portions can make a quick, nutritious breakfast.

Commercial vegetable juices or home-juiced vegetables are a great way to get in several of the 5 to 9 servings of fruits and vegetables recommended daily. If you drink 100% fruit juice, breakfast is certainly the place for it. Remember that fruit sugars are absorbed very quickly into the bloodstream. If combined with a high-fiber breakfast, the juice is absorbed slower. Basal metabolism is higher in the morning than during sleep and increases with exercise. Fruit smoothies (with yogurt, milk, or tofu) and fruit soups (usually contain yogurt) are also creative ways to add to the number of daily fruits and vegetables.

Fruit and vegetables may also be added to breads and quick breads made with whole grain flour, whole wheat pastry flour, or nut flours like almond. Adding flaxseed to baked products adds to the nutritional value (omega-3 fatty acids, phytochemicals, and dietary fiber) without changing taste or consistency.

BREAKFAST ON THE GO!

For many Americans, the problem with breakfast is **time**—time to make it and time to eat it. As already suggested, a slow cooker is a great way to have hot cereals or egg casseroles ready first thing in the morning. Boiled eggs, bananas, apples, pears, grapes, nuts, cheese cubes, vegetable sticks, or a sandwich half can be eaten on the run. Whole grain products, such as bagels, waffles, pancakes, or quick breads, can be put on a plate and covered with plastic wrap the night before; then they will be ready to put into the microwave in the morning and top with peanut butter, fruit, yogurt, cottage cheese, or whatever else sounds yummy. Be creative and make your own *breakfast of champions!*

REMEMBER!

Breakfast is important.

- Eat it—not only because mother said so, but also because the body needs it!
- Breakfast is associated with good health and longevity.
- Eating breakfast improves learning, problem solving, and possibly memory.
- Include foods high in dietary fiber and protein—**not sugar!**
- Any whole foods are breakfast foods—even leftover pizza!
- If in a hurry, grab it and go!

Remember: Breakfast—just eat it!

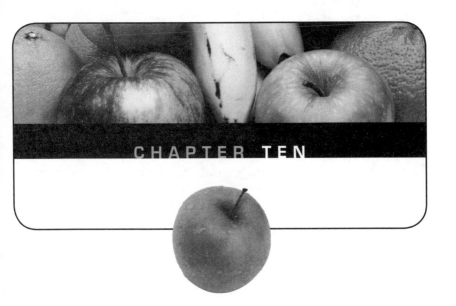

CHAPTER TEN

GETTING OUR
JUST DESSERTS

·

He will eat curds and honey when he knows enough to reject
the wrong and choose the right.
—Isaiah 7:15

The ordinances of the LORD are sure and altogether righteous.
They are...sweeter than honey, than honey from the comb.
—Psalm 19:9–10

SO here we are at the end of the meal. Say this with me please: "There's always room for Jell-O." Isn't that what we were taught? Actually, as Americans, the Constitution does not give us an inalienable right to dessert; but as a nation, we certainly think we do have that right! It's as American as apple pie! The apples we can keep—but we can do a little better with some of the other ingredients.

Some people would be surprised to find out that some cultures have no concept of our supersweet idea of dessert. What a shock! We, too, might do better to think of dessert as fruit, cheese, dark chocolate, or nuts combined with pudding, yogurt, ice cream, fruit ices, or other whole foods. Heavy, sugar-laden desserts have their place, of course. What would birthdays and holidays be without our favorite sweets? However, it is best to think of dessert as a treat instead of a right at every meal.

CHEESE FOR DESSERT?

The idea of a cheese paired with fruit and nuts at the end of a meal might be reminiscent for some of a meal eaten in Europe. A variety of cheeses like a mild cheese, an aged cheese, and a blue cheese might be combined, or just a single one served. Cheeses can be paired with seasonal fruits or dried fruits. Smoked, spiced, or glazed nuts can round out the experience. The great thing about this kind of finish to a meal is that the guests and host or hostess can linger over it and enjoy relaxed conversation—no rush.

Actually, most cheeses contain fewer calories and less fat than a slice of pie. And, as we have discussed, cheese is a good source of protein and calcium. Put it with fruit and nuts, and voilà—a healthy dessert. This kind of course at the end of the meal is a way to encourage the emphasis on quality rather than quantity of food. A little bit goes a long way. This is also another way to get to know the small-production, handmade, artisan cheeses that may be in your area or state. For some ideas for dessert cheeses, read "The Return of the Cheese Course" by Carole Kotkin (available at: *http://www.travellady.com/Issues/Issue81/ 81C-return.htm*).

Always serve cheese at room temperature. Leave cheese wrapped while it's warming up. Allow a 2-ounce portion of each cheese per person.

FRUIT DESSERTS

A variety of fruit breads or puddings may add a healthy end to any meal. One easy way to include fresh fruit as a dessert is by making a fruit bread or pudding in a slow cooker. This may be topped with other fruit, nuts, pudding, ice cream, or whipped cream. Even simpler, just cut up whatever fruit is on hand, toss with a little orange juice to keep it from oxidizing, add honey to taste, and dash on vanilla flavoring, cinnamon, or nutmeg—that makes an instant, fresh, nutritious dessert with whole fresh fruit! To sauté or panfry the fruit, just choose a fresh fruit and cook with butter or add butter at the end. Top with homemade muesli or granola. Other ways to use fruit for dessert would be grilling, poaching, or baking. Heating fruit brings out the natural sugars. Honey may be added after cooking for extra sweetness. Topping fruit desserts with cream, whipped cream, ice cream, or yogurt just adds to its nutritional value and richness. For an opposite approach, dairy desserts may be topped with fresh or canned fruit.

USE HONEY, HONEY

Honey, a natural sweetener used for thousands of years, is rich in vitamins, minerals, and antioxidants. The darker the honey, the more nutritional value it has. A few things should be kept in mind when using honey instead of sugar in cooking. Use about half as much honey as the sugar called for in the recipe. Also, reduce the amount of liquid in the recipe by 20% or one-fifth. For example, if a recipe calls for 2 cups of sugar, substitute 1 cup of honey. Reduce the liquid called for by approximately ¼ cup for each cup of honey used. Add ½ teaspoon baking soda for each cup of honey used. If honey is used in the recipe, reduce the oven temperature by 25°F to prevent overbrowning.

CHOCOLATE IS A GOOD THING

Would life be worth living without chocolate? Discussing this could be a complete book in itself. Sitting through the movie

Chocolate is enough to reveal that chocolate is what life is all about…well, almost. And then seeing *Willy Wonka* [and *Charlie*] *and the Chocolate Factory*…. Need I say more? The lure of chocolate is powerful. Chocolate is made from cacao beans, which have powerful nutrients and phytochemicals and have been used for thousands of years by indigenous tribes in Central and South America for snake bites, parasites, and a general anesthetic. Chocolate has always been used as a stimulant. Recent research has shown that the nutritional benefits of dark chocolate, in particular, can reduce the risks of heart disease, stroke, and cancer.

However, more than for disease prevention, we want chocolate because it makes us feel good! Debra Waterhouse, a registered dietitian and the author of the book *Why Women Need Chocolate*, thinks both culture and chemicals attract us to chocolate. Chemicals in chocolate affect levels of serotonin and endorphins in the body, which relax and calm us, reducing stress and anxiety. Chocolate also raises the body's level of phenylethylamine, which the body releases in response to romance! No wonder it makes us euphoric. Chocolate has it all—if eaten in moderation, of course.

Effects of other foods on mood have long been observed, too. Food can increase feelings of happiness, contentment, and alertness, as well as feelings of depression, anxiety, failure, and guilt. The reasons for these effects are complex and include not only the nutritional and pharmacological substances in the foods themselves, but differences in the people who consume them.

Desserts, however, seem to put most people in a very jolly if not positively ecstatic mood. Reasons for this transition go further than just the chocolate. We could include the ample amounts of carbohydrate (starch and sugar) included in most typical desserts. These ingredients cause the brain to release the chemicals that cause a natural high, euphoria, increased energy, and all those things related to being happy, happy, happy! However, if we get too great a dose at any one time, we eventually crash. Cakes, cookies, and fudge are known as pleasure foods not only because they delight the taste buds, but also because they can bring on a calm and happy feeling—at least temporarily.

This sugar-induced sense of euphoria comes from several chemical mechanisms in the brain. First of all, the sheer pleasure of tasting a chocolate treat or powdery doughnut stimulates the brain's pleasure pathways and the release of serotonin, dopamine, and endorphins, the chemical causes of that good feeling. Also a quick surge of energy is experienced as the sugar hits the bloodstream. Unfortunately, that energized feeling lasts only as long as the sugar rush. Once blood sugar levels drop (about an hour or two later), a feeling of being drained and out of sorts is what is left. It is easy to become an addict looking for another hit. Excessive insulin from too much refined flour and sugar can also lead to higher triglycerides, higher cholesterol, poor HDL to LDL ratios, higher blood pressure, excess fat production and storage, obesity, insulin resistance, and dramatically increased risk for diabetes, heart disease, and stroke.

ADDICTS, TAKE NOTE

Carbohydrate (starch and sugar) can be as addictive as any drug, and the addiction is real!

Let's say then, that a little sugar goes a long way. We can accomplish decreased exposure to that addictive agent by eating smaller portions than usual of our favorite dessert or simply eating healthier desserts!

Also know that stress causes cravings for those feel-good foods like chocolate and carbohydrates. The answer to such cravings is to "eat responsibly"—keeping blood sugar up with regular healthy meals and snacks, if need be. Moderate amounts of sugar eaten with meals are burned for energy just like any other carbohydrate. The key is to eat mixed meals that blunt insulin spikes and, of course, to get enough physical activity to burn off calories eaten. A colleague of mine at the university where I teach makes every Monday "Dessert Night" at his house. What a great way to teach his children that desserts and sweets are a special treat, not an everyday provision.

REAL SUGAR

Well, we have to talk about it—the "s" word. Sugar, as discussed in relation to carbohydrates, is simple—it is absorbed very fast into the blood during digestion. We don't need to demonize it again, but we do need to recognize that sugar can hardly be avoided in our world. We can make a conscious effort to limit it, but it will always be there to lure us.

An average American eats between 100 and 160 pounds of sugar a year! Does that sound impossible? There are about 10 teaspoons or 40 grams of sugar in one 12-ounce soft drink. Drinking one 12-ounce soft drink a day for 365 days equals 36 pounds of sugar a year. If that were all the sugar eaten in a day, that would be within the recommendations of not more than about 10% of daily calories from refined sugar. However, sugar intake does not stop there. Most Americans eat and drink at least twice that much a day. Almost every processed food contains sugar in some form. It's in everything—chicken soup, pickles, pork and beans, peanut butter, bread, macaroni and cheese, mustard, relish, yogurt, canned fruit and vegetables, salad dressings, and more. Ketchup is one-third sugar, for heaven's sake!

Reducing sugar from everyday life is not easy. One of the best ways to limit the sweet life is to not drink it! Also, as we have said before, whole natural foods are best. When we purchase processed foods, we **must** read the labels. Honey, molasses, maple syrup, fruit juices, raw sugar, cane juice, brown sugar, maple sugar, natural fruit preserves, and stevia are all natural sweeteners that can be used in moderation. We will never get away from refined sugar, but we can monitor it. And we especially need to stay away from HFCS—remember that bad stuff?

SUGAR SUBSTITUTES

The FDA has approved these five sugar substitutes:

- Saccharine (Sweet'N Low)
- Acesulfame-K (Sunett)
- Neotame
- Sucralose (Splenda)
- Aspartame (NutraSweet or Equal), used in Crystal Light, diet sodas, chewing gum, and toothpaste

Although the FDA says that they are all safe, they are **not** natural. Neotame is the newest and sweetest of the approved sugar substitutes. It is approximately 7,000 times sweeter than sugar, so a very small amount is used to sweeten products. Splenda is currently one of the most advertised sugar substitutes; one advantage for this substitute is the ability to cook with Splenda. Aspartame seems to create the most problems with side effects. There is a warning on the label for anyone who has an inborn error of metabolism called phenylketonuria (PKU); these people should not eat aspartame. Long-term effects of using aspartame, especially for pregnant women and children, are yet to be determined. These artificial sweeteners are found in thousands of products, so read labels.

SUGAR ALCOHOLS

Sugar alcohols are ingredients used as sweeteners and bulking agents. They occur naturally in foods and come from plant products, such as fruits and berries. As a sugar substitute, they provide fewer calories (about a half to one-third fewer calories) than regular sugar. This is because they are converted to glucose more slowly, require little or no insulin to be metabolized, and don't cause sudden increases in blood sugar. This makes them popular among individuals with diabetes. Their use is becoming more common. Sugar alcohols like mannitol, sorbitol, and xylitol do not cause tooth decay like sugar does. Therefore, many sugar-free gums are made with sugar alcohols. Sugar alcohols also add texture to foods, retain moisture better, and prevent foods from browning when they are heated.

STEVIA

As far as natural noncaloric sweeteners go, stevia is the only product available. However, in the United States, the FDA calls it a dietary supplement and not a sweetener. Stevia is a noncaloric herb native to Paraguay that has been used for centuries in South America and for more than 25 years in Japan as a sweetener and flavor enhancer. Even though you probably won't find it in supermarkets, most health food stores in the US carry it.

This herbal substance has been used safely for hundreds of years, is in almost half of all sweetened foods consumed in Japan, has been cultivated and studied extensively around the world with no reports of any ill side effects, and has the ability to prevent tooth decay, inhibit the growth of certain bacteria, balance blood sugar levels, heal wounds, and actually **reduce the craving for sweets**, not increase it!

The bottom line on sugar and sugar substitutes is this: **they are not whole natural foods**. In the Big Picture, **a little** refined sugar (16 calories per teaspoon) is a much lesser evil that **a lot** of artificial sugar. Some evidence suggests that artificial sweeteners increase the craving for more sweets, just as sugar does.

A SHORT HISTORY OF SUGAR

When the process of purification of sucrose was first invented centuries ago, it was carried out by hand and only small quantities of table sugar could be made. It was so expensive, only royalty and other very rich people could afford to eat it on a regular basis. Degenerative diseases from refined carbohydrates were once the privilege of only the rich. Even 100 years ago, with sugar used moderately in home baking, desserts were balanced with healthy whole foods. Now, processed commercial foods full of sugar are available at every turn. We don't even have to get out of our car. And now everyone can afford them. Let's take a look at something Ethel Renwick wrote in 1976:

We eat more candy than eggs; we eat more sugar than vegetables, fruits, and eggs put together; we drink more soft drinks than milk; and beginning in 1971 we started eating more processed foods than fresh. We do not have to be nutritionists to know that this is a downhill race we are in; unless we make a drastic change, we are leading our children and grandchildren to a higher incidence of degenerative diseases than our present deplorable rate. I think our problem is that we have not added up our diet. We think a little sugar here and there, a soft drink now and then, a little additive to a food, and "enriched" flour cannot hurt. But that is not realistic. **Refined foods, sugar, and additives are in almost everything we eat.** We talk about bringing up our children in a good Christian home! What we mean is that we have looked after two-thirds of our responsibility to the best of our ability. But we have left out the other third—an abundance of God's provisions for the bodies of which we are stewards.

—Ethel H. Renwick, *Let's Try Real Food* (bold added)

My goodness! And that was 30 years ago. Look what progress we have made. In the last 30 years, obesity, heart disease, stroke, and diabetes have more than doubled in the United States, and these same diseases are now a worldwide epidemic. Oops, I really didn't mean to preach in the dessert chapter, but look where a little refined flour and sugar (and hydrogenated oils) have taken us. What started out as an extravagance—a rare treat, a weekly homemade delight—has gotten way out of hand.

Around the world, people in all cultures have been using sugar responsibly **at home** for centuries. It was not until the commercially available processed foods with excess sugar and hydrogenated fats flooded the world market that the worldwide obesity epidemic began.

One response to the global explosion of fast foods was the Slow Food Movement, started in the 1980s, which was created to celebrate local foods and their traditions. And that includes wonderful homemade desserts!

We can look at how our own bodies respond to sugar or sugar substitutes and make our own judgment about eating them. We are individually responsible for what goes into our mouths—it is our decision and our choice. Most of us can eat sweets and desserts in **moderation** and maintain adequate physical activity, but some people just cannot. Some may have to go off sugar cold turkey. For great reading about reducing sugar consumption, try these books:

- *Sugar Blues* by William Dufty
- *Get the Sugar Out: 501 Simple Ways to Cut the Sugar in Any Diet* by Ann Louise Gittleman
- *The New Sugar Busters! Cut Sugar to Trim Fat* by H. Leighton Steward (See also *www.sugarbusters.com.*)

OUR RESPONSIBILITY

Whatever we do, it is up to us to be the hope for the generations to come. I'm not being melodramatic. If parents and grandparents don't take a stand for healthy living, then who will? We have to make common sense common practice once again. If you or your children can't cook, learn together. Enroll in a cooking class. Buy a cookbook and just start cooking! Watch the Food Network. If this generation doesn't do something, there will be no recipes to hand down to the next!

My favorite food magazine is *Saveur*. I wait for my monthly edition with bated breath. I took my dog-eared copy of the issue featuring Cuban cuisine with me to Cuba. I always consult the Web site *www.saveur.com* before I take any trip. *Saveur* magazine, as do other culinary publications (*Gourmet, Bon Appetit, Cook's Illustrated, Taste of the South,* and others), celebrate local, traditional cuisine from around the world. As I looked in a recent issue of *Saveur* at a recipe from Sorrento, Italy, for lemon custard made with local Sorrento lemons, I could almost feel the Italian sunshine coming through the recipe!

My parents grow blueberries and, through the years, have accumulated several traditional blueberry dessert recipes that are unique and special to us. These recipes are being passed down. Passing down the recipe box from one generation to the next may be more important than realized. Some of our most vivid memories of childhood and love come from familiar and comforting aromas in the kitchen. Wonderful traditional desserts, among other recipes, are personal treasures for a family and national treasures for a culture. We must not lose them to the drive-through and frozen food case!

HEALTHY DESSERTS

Isn't healthy dessert an oxymoron? Actually, no. Just take the Italians, for example. My daughter spent a year in Torino, Italy, as a nanny for an Italian couple with two small children. In addition to the normal end of a meal, which was fruit and cheese or yogurt, for special occasions, custards, puddings, panna cotta, tiramisu, and other milk- or cream-based desserts were common. Of course, it wouldn't be Italy without gelato and fruit ices. Typical pies, pastries, and cookies are enjoyed in Italy, but these are also usually eaten only on special occasions.

For an assortment of milk-based desserts, review these books:

- *Gelato! Italian Ice Creams, Sorbetti & Granite* by Pamela Sheldon Johns
- *The Splendid Spoonful: From Custard to Crème Brûlée* by Barbara Lauterbach
- *Elegantly Easy Crème Brûlée & Other Custard Desserts* by Debbie Puente

Most cultures have their version of custards, puddings, or yogurts. A popular Spanish and Latin American dessert with many variations is flan, or quesillo in Venezuela. In the American South, family recipes for rice pudding, banana pudding, bread pudding, egg custard, and trifle (adapted from the English) have been handed down for generations. Making desserts that are milk-based adds to the nutritional value of a meal. Topping fresh or stewed fruit with yogurt, pudding, or cream makes a fast, nutritious dessert. Adding natural fruit preserves to sweeten plain whole yogurt is an excellent, nutrient-dense dessert. Using leftover rice for pudding is healthy and economical. Check your favorite cookbook for a rice pudding recipe, or do a Web search for a variety of options. Remember that rice pudding, like oatmeal, can be cooked overnight in a slow cooker for a healthy and delicious breakfast (or dessert!).

Speaking of oats, this breakfast favorite also makes great desserts. What's better than the smell of oatmeal cookies baking? Many a fruit crisp or cobbler has been topped with oatmeal. Oatmeal cake is a moist and healthy choice for dessert or breakfast coffee cake. Recipes for healthy oatmeal and other whole grain cakes and desserts can be found in *More-with-Less Cookbook* by Doris Longacre.

Other desserts that can be healthy are Italian cheesecake and panna cotta. Using ricotta cheese for the cheesecake makes it a high-protein dessert that is loaded with calcium, magnesium, and selenium. Panna cotta is another Italian dairy dessert that is brimming with nutrition and flavor. Add any fresh fruit topping to increase the nutritional value of each. Both are rich, so small servings are sufficient. Again, go to the Web and find a variety of ricotta cheesecake or panna cotta recipes.

HEALTHY DESSERT INGREDIENTS

Sometimes for dessert, our family members just have a handful of chocolate chips and pecans. Keep plenty of ingredients for healthy desserts on hand. Here are some ideas:

- **Grains:** Whole wheat pastry flour, rolled oats, rye flakes, wheat flakes, rolled barley, brown rice flakes, cracked wheat, millet, buckwheat
- **Dairy:** Milk, cream, half-and-half, yogurt, frozen yogurt, ice cream
- **Seeds:** Sesame, sunflower, flax, pumpkin

- **Nuts:** Walnuts, almonds, cashews, pecans, hazelnuts, coconut, pistachios
- **Sweeteners:** Honey, molasses, maple syrup, fruit juices, raw sugar, cane juice, brown sugar, maple sugar, natural fruit preserves, stevia
- **Flavorings:** Semisweet chocolate chips, vanilla extract, almond extract, grated citrus rinds, cinnamon, ginger
- **Fats:** Naturally pressed oils (olive, almond, sesame, peanut), butter, coconut oil
- **Fresh fruits:** Apples, pears, bananas—whatever is in season
- **Dried fruits:** Dried apples, raisins, berries, figs, dates

REMEMBER!

Be not deceived about desserts:

- Although we have concentrated on healthy desserts in this chapter, traditional desserts occasionally may be part of healthy eating...if eater is willing to exercise off the extra calories.

- Do not use shortening, margarine, or refined/hydrogenated oils in desserts. Real butter, lard, or healthy unrefined plant oils are always a better choice.

- Desserts can be healthy, but **we** have to make them that way!

Remember: Think of dessert as a treat or special occasion— not a right at every meal.

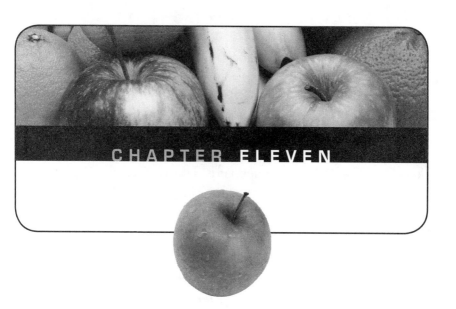

CHAPTER ELEVEN

SNACKS FOR GRAZERS

———————●———————

In those days John the Baptist came, preaching in the Desert of Judea....
This is he who was spoken of through the prophet Isaiah....
John's clothes were made of camel's hair, and he had a leather belt
around his waist. His food was locusts and wild honey.
—Matthew 3:1, 3–4

WE may not share John the Baptist's taste in dress or snack food, but he had the right idea! Snacking has and always will be with us. Most every culture has its own idea of what to eat between meals. It may be another meal! Eating several small meals a day is common in many countries.

We Americans have a tendency to bring out a tasty, but not-so-healthy, treat if the preacher comes to call or the in-laws come by for a visit or the next-door neighbors drop by for coffee. And, of course, nothing says "doughnuts" like Sunday School!

However, that doesn't necessarily have to be the case. We can be prepared to serve healthy snacks to our family and friends if we keep healthy foods in our cupboards. This is especially important for our own families and a **must** for our grandchildren.

Keep the pantry, refrigerator, and freezer stocked with good things, and keep some colorful, inviting, healthy foods in plain sight on the counter.

In the Pantry

- Canned beans and peas
- Whole grain breads, crackers, cereals
- Wheat bran
- Pasta
- Tomato and vegetable pasta sauces
- Tomato and vegetable juices
- Rice
- Canned sardines, tuna, and salmon
- Canned fruit in juice or light syrup, applesauce
- Dried fruit
- Canned vegetables
- Canned nuts and seeds, roasted peanuts in the shell
- Nonrefined, naturally pressed, extra-virgin olive, peanut, avocado, walnut, and flax oils
- Sweet potatoes, onions, and garlic
- Honey

In the Refrigerator

- Cheese
- Eggs
- Butter
- Natural nut butters
- Organic dairy products (milk, cream, yogurt, kefir, buttermilk)
- Tofu
- Sliced deli meats (turkey, ham)
- 100% fruit juice
- Fresh vegetables (carrots, red and green peppers, broccoli, celery, mushrooms, zucchini)
- Leafy vegetables (red- and green-leaf lettuce, romaine, and spinach)

In the Freezer

- Extra whole grain bread
- Whole grain pancake and muffin mix
- Wheat germ
- Frozen vegetables and fruits (berries especially)
- Meat, poultry, and fish
- Nuts in packages
- Organic ice cream and frozen yogurt

On the Counter

- Bananas
- Apples
- Oranges
- Tangerines
- Tomatoes
- Whatever looks yummy at the market and is in season!

Snacking has become a favorite American pastime. However, many of the foods Americans think of as snack foods are junk foods (empty calories), unfortunately! So we need to pay better attention to snacks we provide our family.

Snacking is a very important part of a child's everyday diet. During this important growth period in the life cycle, children expend much more energy in activity and development in relation to their size than do adults. However, their tiny tummies are too small to hold very much food at one time. Healthy snacks help round out the daily nutritional requirements of children and provide as much as one-fourth of their caloric needs.

Sometimes in our busy lives, we struggle to find time to sit down with our families for even **one** meal a day, so to maintain a nutritious diet, snacks should be a planned part of healthy eating. Adults model eating habits for their children and grandchildren, and this certainly applies to snacks. If the pantry is filled with empty-calorie snacks, the whole family eats empty calories! If adults in the family eat and enjoy nutritious snacks as well as nutritious meals, that example encourages the children to develop healthy eating habits for a lifetime. Children of all ages are more interested in eating healthy snacks if they help pick them out while shopping (especially fruits and vegetables). Although grocery shopping with children can be a challenge, it can also be a great learning experience. Older children can begin learning simple cooking techniques by helping prepare their own snacks with supervision.

So what makes a good snack? A good snack is **nutrient dense** (the most nutrients with the least calories). A good snack is a whole food. A good snack has plenty of dietary fiber. A good snack has healthy fats. A good snack is colorful. A good snack provides calcium. A good snack always includes protein. Snacks are a great way to help provide a portion of the 25 to 30 grams of dietary fiber, five to nine servings of fruits and vegetables, and three to four servings of dairy foods that adults need per day. Let's consider a few age-appropriate recommendations.

Toddlers and preschoolers: When planning snacks for this age, think small. Also avoid foods that are hard or round that might cause choking—like nuts, seeds, popcorn, dried fruits, and raw vegetables. Cut up meat, hot dogs, grapes, or cherry tomatoes. Spread peanut butter thin or dilute with applesauce or pureed fruit.

Children: School-age children begin choosing and/or preparing their own snacks. Avoid falling for and buying every advertised snack the child begs to have. Make sure snacks are simple, tasty, and healthy. Read labels carefully. Designate an area in the refrigerator and pantry for healthy snacks.

Adolescents and teens: On average, teens probably eat more snacks than regular meals daily. That means it is important to pack the backpack with healthy snack choices to be munched on throughout the day. That way they won't have to grab food from a vending machine or fast-food restaurant before or after activities. However, healthy choices can be made no matter where a teen is.

Adults: Just call them dashboard diners. Surveys have shown that more than 90% of adults admit to eating often or occasionally while driving. The National Highway Traffic Safety Administration put together a list of the worst foods to eat while driving. In general, these are foods that are drippy, sticky, or greasy or liquids in an open container.

Older adults: Older adults who are less active and who burn fewer calories may actually feel more comfortable eating several small meals a day—in other words, lots of snacks! Snacks should be carefully planned to make sure every snack is nutrient dense so that no calories are wasted. A bedtime snack of a food with the sleep-inducing amino acid tryptophan helps some restless seniors get a better night's sleep. Here is a short list of such snacks:

- Dairy products like ice cream, yogurt or kefir, warm milk, or buttermilk
- Crackers and cheese
- Whole grain cereal with milk
- Oatmeal or oatmeal cookies with milk
- Natural nut butters in a sandwich or with crackers and milk
- Boiled egg or scrambled egg with cheese
- Pasta, olive oil, butter, and Parmesan cheese with chopped chicken or turkey

SNACK IDEAS FOR ALL AGES

- Whole grain bread sandwich with lean meats, poultry, tuna fish, or cheese
- Corn chips (especially blue) with bean dip
- Whole grain cereal, loose or mixed with yogurt
- Homemade whole grain cereal bar
- Homemade whole grain or vegetable muffin
- Popcorn plain or topped with grated cheese
- Bean burrito
- Bean or cheese quesadilla or nachos with salsa
- Raw vegetables with olive oil, yogurt, or cottage cheese dip
- Grape tomatoes
- Cottage cheese with fresh fruit or vegetables
- Pudding
- Kefir or drinkable yogurt
- Baked sweet potato (whole or sliced)
- Hard-boiled egg
- Apple slices with cheese, nuts, or seeds
- Whole wheat pita and hummus

- Nuts with dried fruit
- Shake or smoothie with milk or yogurt and fresh fruit
- Frozen fruit slices
- Thin-crust or whole wheat crust pizza
- Whole wheat waffle with fresh fruit
- Homemade soup, stew, or chili
- Almost anything with natural peanut butter or other nut butters

For additional calcium and protein, include milk, flavored milk, drinkable yogurt, or kefir with snacks when possible. **Remember: Leftovers of any healthy foods are great brown-bag and snack choices.**

WHEN TO SNACK

Scheduled times. For toddlers, preschoolers, and children, offer snacks at regular times according to their daily schedules. Avoid unlimited snacking. Whatever the age, don't plan snacks too close to mealtime. A good rule of thumb is to eat a light meal or snack every three to four hours. Avoid snacking on sticky or chewy foods that might contribute to tooth decay. Fibrous foods like apples and celery actually help clean the teeth!

Remember that dietary fiber, good fats, and protein provide satiety or a feeling of fullness after we eat. They also help slow down the absorption of simple carbohydrates like starches or sugars that are eaten at the same time. A snack after aerobic or strengthening exercise should include complex carbohydrate and protein for muscle replenishing and building tissue.

Brown-bag it. Snacking is not just for kids, and brown bagging isn't either! More and more of us take our lunch (and snacks) with us as we leave for school or work each day. That means that desktop dining, locker lunches, and study snacks need to be not only nutritious but also safe. Make sure food and containers are clean. Keep cold foods cold and hot foods hot. Use a vacuum bottle, insulated lunch box with freezer pack, or freeze a drink or water bottle to include in the lunch bag. If a microwave is available, make sure hot foods are hot before eating. A cheery note in the brown bag is nice too!

Teatime. That singularly British institution has made a comeback across the big pond! It may be said that afternoon tea is the king (or queen) of snacks. Although decidedly less fancy on a daily basis than in Great Britain, afternoon tea American-style can be healthy, as well as fun for the family. Teatime with whole wheat sandwiches (cream cheese and cucumber, egg salad, and/or tomato), scones made with whole wheat baking mix or whole wheat pastry flour, oatmeal cookies, and/or fresh fruit with whipped cream, properly served along with hot tea with cream, of course, is a wonderful activity; children can help prepare, serve, and enjoy eating these snacks with parents, grandparents, and/or friends.

REMEMBER!

Keep in mind these snacking tips:

- Keep a good supply of healthy snack foods in the home.
- Include a source of dietary fiber, protein, and/or healthy fats in every snack.
- Use snack time to add healthy dairy products to daily intake.
- Make snacks age appropriate.

Remember: Snacks are really minimeals. Make them work for your family and you as part of a healthy-eating lifestyle!

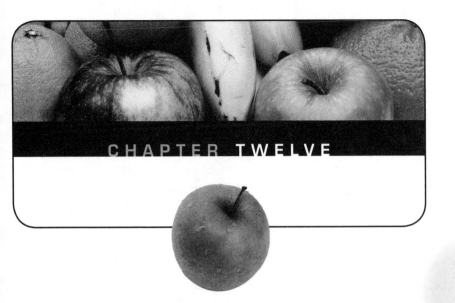

CHAPTER TWELVE

MAKE CALORIES COUNT

●

The king assigned [the young men] a daily amount of food and
wine from the king's table.... But Daniel resolved not to defile
himself with the royal food and wine.
—Daniel 1:5, 8

EMPTY calories versus nutrient-dense calories—what does that mean anyway? Think of it as 1 cup of a sugared soft drink versus 1 cup of low-fat milk. Both have about 100 calories, but the cola has zero nutrients. The milk contributes 3% of the average daily adult need for folic acid and vitamin C, 8% of thiamin, 11% of potassium, 16% of protein and vitamin A, 24% of riboflavin, and 30% of calcium! Now that is nutrient density! Nutrient density is the amount of nutrients in a food relative to the amount of calories. The higher level of nutrients and the fewer number of calories, the more nutrient dense the food is.

SOFT DRINKS, THE EMPTIEST OF CALORIES

Overweight and obesity have doubled in the United States in the last 20 years, and it is not surprising that these statistics paralleled the increase in consumption of sugared soft drinks. The results of several national self-reported food surveys have shown that **many nutrient-rich foods have been replaced by sugared soft drinks and fruit drinks**. In fact, in the last 20 years, sugared soft drink consumption has increased by 300%. It has been shown that for each 12-ounce sugared soft drink consumed daily, the risk of obesity is increased by 60%. Sweetened drinks are a particular problem since the empty calories are ingested in liquid form and are easily overconsumed. These calories not only replace nutrient-dense foods, but also provide additional caloric load. One study reported that it was not uncommon for teenagers to get 500 to 1,000 calories per day from sugar-sweetened drinks.

BEWARE OF HIGH-FRUCTOSE CORN SYRUP

High-fructose corn syrup (HFCS) now represents more than 40% of the sweeteners in foods and beverages in the US. It is the major caloric sweetener in sugared soft drinks, fruit drinks, sports drinks, and teas. The huge array of HFCS-sweetened food products includes ketchup, yogurt, cereals, baked goods, gum, jams, and jellies. Fat-free products may contain an inordinate amount. Some research suggests that HFCS may be digested and metabolized differently in the body than sucrose, causing even more significant weight gain. Though these findings may be preliminary, HFCS is, nonetheless, a major hidden source of empty calories in many foods.

BE SURE THE JUICE IS JUICE

What about fruit juice? The word **juice** is the key. When shopping for juice, be sure that the label says "100% fruit juice with no added sugar," and not "fruit drink." Even 100% juice is high in natural sugars. The American Academy of Pediatrics recommends that children limit daily amounts of juice to about a cup or less a day and be encouraged to eat whole fruits instead. Most juices are enriched with vitamin C, and some are fortified with calcium. However, many nutrients, such as water-soluble vitamins, minerals, dietary fiber, and phytochemicals, are lost in the processing of juices. The skins, pulp, and seeds of whole fruits contain much of their nutritional value.

Vegetable juices are excellent choices for beverages since they are very nutrient dense (low in calories and high in nutritional value). Some people may want or need to choose the low-sodium varieties. Try V8 V.Fusion for a full serving of both fruit *and* vegetable in an 8-ounce glass! Remember to keep vegetable and fruit juices tightly closed and return them to the refrigerator immediately after every use to preserve nutrients.

GOOD AND BAD ALTERNATIVES

Analysis of diets in children and adolescents has shown that when flavored milk, yogurt, ice cream, and pudding are chosen instead of sugar-sweetened beverages, vitamins and minerals increase and total fat, saturated fat, and total sugars decrease. Even though these dairy foods have added sugar, they contain much less than the sugared beverages they are replacing. The American Academy of Pediatrics recommends that the sale of sweetened drinks be restricted in schools. Some schools are already replacing sweetened beverages with water, milk, and 100% juices. Weight-conscious teens should be aware of the research that links milk with weight reduction as a part of a lower-calorie diet. Choosing low-fat and fat-free milk products might also help raise the intake of calcium—and when calcium intake increases, so does the intake of other important vitamins and minerals.

As stated before, the gourmet coffee drinks adults and students love can pack a fattening punch! Whether hot or iced, a large coffee combined with sugar, sugar syrups, whole milk, or whipped cream can deliver up to 600 calories, 25 grams of fat, and 100 grams of carbohydrates. Regular coffee, tea, and cocoa, however, are excellent beverage choices, calorie-wise. Coffee, cocoa, and black or green teas (even decaffeinated) contain phytochemicals that are not bound by adding milk.

Although sugared beverages are the ultimate empty-calorie food, many other foods are not far behind. Usually, solid foods that are high in sugar are also high in fat—especially baked goods. Other junk foods may be high in fat and salt. Some may combine processed flours or starch with sugar and/or salt. The common denominator is that all are high in calories and low in nutritional value.

POWER FOODS

The ultimate nutrient-dense foods are what some consider "power foods." Power foods pack in the most nutrients per calorie. These include, but are not limited to, the following:

- **Nuts, seeds, olives, and their natural oils:** peanuts, almonds, walnuts, Brazil nuts, hazelnuts, sesame seeds, flaxseeds
- **Red, yellow, orange, and blue fruits and vegetables:** apples, tomatoes, watermelon, berries, oranges, kiwifruit, sweet and chili peppers, grapes, sweet potatoes, pumpkin, mangoes, butternut squash
- **Cruciferous and green vegetables:** spinach, kale, broccoli, watercress, greens, bok choy, brussels sprouts, cabbage, cauliflower, avocados
- **Whole grains:** especially oatmeal and quinoa
- **Beans and peas:** black beans, kidney beans, yellow split peas, chickpeas, lentils
- **Wild fatty fish:** sardines, wild salmon, tuna
- **Onions, garlic, and mushrooms**
- **Soy:** edamame, miso, tempeh
- **Dairy products:** especially fermented; for example, yogurt
- **Tea:** especially green tea

Power foods—superfoods or "the world's healthiest foods"— provide the most bang for your buck! Check out these resources for power foods: *www.whfoods.com* and *Superfoods Rx* by Steven Pratt and Kathy Matthews.

REMEMBER!

When taking in calories, make them count.

- Avoid sugared drinks that provide empty calories.
- Drink milk, which provides close to the same number of calories as same amount of sugared drink but is packed with nutrients.
- Buy fruit and vegetable juice that is real juice: 100% juice with no added sugar, not fruit drink.
- Make calories count by eating nutrient-dense power foods.

Remember: Make empty calories the exception, not the rule. Save them for special occasions or a "treat" time!

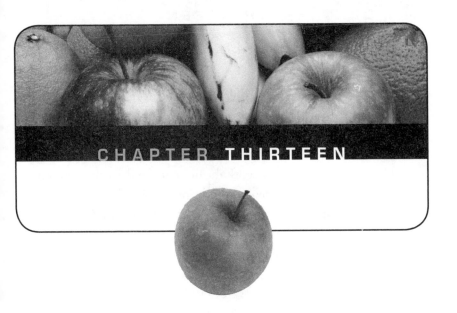

HONEY, I ATE THE WHOLE THING

Listen, my son, and be wise, and keep your heart on the right path.
Do not join those who drink too much wine or gorge themselves on
meat, for drunkards and gluttons become poor.
—Proverbs 23:19–21

ALTHOUGH I have heard sermons against drinking a single drop of wine many times from the pulpit, I have yet to hear a sermon about eating a 36-ounce steak. Yet gluttony is a real problem in America today. Of course, I'm not saying that eating in itself is bad. We have already established that the world is full of good things that God has blessed us with, and food is certainly one of those good things. However, it is possible to become so caught up in a pleasure, whether food or drink or sex or work or possessions, that we can no longer enjoy other things and would be willing to sacrifice other pleasures for the one. This could be called an addiction, dependency, or weakness. Unhealthy living, whether it is eating junk food, being a couch potato, or being a workaholic, can lead to the altered metabolism, hormone imbalance, altered brain chemistry, and other body dysfunctions related to loss of self-control. God does not give us a top-ten ranking for overindulgences because *any* good gift can become sin.

Overindulgence, as in gluttony and drunkenness, are part of the sinful nature that Paul describes in Galatians 5 (vv. 19–21), but the fruit of the Spirit, he goes on to say, *"is love, joy, peace, patience, kindness, goodness, faithfulness, gentleness and **self-control*** (vv. 22–23, bold added). We all have our own weaknesses and obsessions—be it sugar, salt, alcohol, sports, shopping, work, sex, the Internet, or TV. None of us can point a finger at the other. We (because of our sinful nature) have trouble practicing self-control alone. Whatever our indulgences, vices, or addictions, the only answer is self-control through the work of the Holy Spirit in us. We can begin to practice healthy living by learning **moderation in all things** and when to **just say no.**

God's blessing of an abundance of food and drink is to be enjoyed and celebrated! He wants us to take the time to savor all the colors, aromas, tastes, and textures. He gives us those wonderful gifts because He loves us. But we are not good stewards if we abuse anything He provides for us. Unfortunately, in the last 30 years especially, we have increasingly abused whole natural food by overrefining, overprocessing, and reinventing what we eat.

SLOW FOOD

Yes, we are what we eat or drink. Sadly, as a nation, we have found that eating supersized portions of refined and processed foods devoid of nutrition, for the most part, has contributed to the current epidemic of obesity.

Picture the millions of Americans in their cars at the drive-through to pick up their fast food that they gulp down while rushing to the next appointment. Now think of a long, relaxing meal in Italy, France, or Greece, where time is taken to actually savor the flavors of freshly prepared local food. There is a world of difference in what is considered "fast food" and "slow food." We all know what fast food is. However, our parents or grandparents may have to tell some of us what slow food is. Whether made completely from scratch or not, food that is made with love and attention and recipes that are shared with others demand time to really taste and enjoy what is being eaten.

An International Slow Food Movement began in Italy to protest the first fast-food restaurant in Rome. Now with members on five continents, Slow Food celebrates the enjoyment of food, the preservation of regional foods, culinary traditions, and small producers. Research shows that in countries where taste and enjoyment of food is important, portion sizes of food in restaurants, in supermarkets, and at home are much smaller than Americans would expect. In fact, in France the portion sizes for typical restaurant entrées are estimated to be more than 50% smaller than American entrées.

My dad would say that the way to lose weight is to "just close your mouth." When we slow down the eating process, our bodies are better able to tell us just when to do that—close our mouths. It takes about 20 minutes for us to feel full after we start eating. Most of the time, we eat so fast that we are way past full and up to miserable by 20 minutes. If we eat smaller portions more slowly and actually relish each bite, we just might end up eating less, but enjoying it more!

SERVING SIZES

Actually, it is the portion size of our meals and not serving sizes of our food that has increased. A portion of food is defined by the USDA as "the amount of food you choose to eat." A serving of food is defined as "a standard amount used to help give advice about how much to eat or to identify how many calories and nutrients are in a food." Serving sizes for US food guides have been essentially the same since they were introduced in the 1940s. It is just that most Americans either don't know or don't care what serving sizes of foods are. Food labels all have nutritional facts that include serving size and servings per container. However, the serving size on some labels may be a portion size rather than a standard serving size.

For example, an average portion of meat is 2 or 3 ounces; however, one serving is 1 ounce. Therefore, a 36-ounce prime rib special would be 12 portions or 36 servings! This is enough meat for a week or two. Restaurant portion sizes have increased quite obviously in the last 20 to 30 years. Restaurant plate and glass sizes have also increased to be able to hold it all. Research has shown that a person eats more without realizing it as portion sizes increase. With loaded baked potatoes the size of footballs, half-gallon drinks, and cookies the size of Frisbees, it's easy to see how Americans overeat. Even when healthy foods are eaten, the amounts of those foods are also important. One serving of cooked oatmeal is *not* whatever fits into the big cereal bowl.

The following guidelines help in visualizing **one standard serving** (not portion) for most food guides.

Whole Grain Cereal, Bread, Rice, and Pasta
- 1 slice of bread (half of a regular-sized hamburger bun or bagel)
- 1 cup of dry cereal
- ½ cup of cooked cereal, rice, or pasta

Vegetables and Fruits
- 2 cups of raw leafy vegetables
- 1 cup of other vegetables, cooked or raw
- 1 cup of cooked dried beans or peas (one vegetable serving)

- 1 cup of tofu (one vegetable serving)
- 1 cup of vegetable juice or fruit juice
- 1 medium apple, banana, orange, or other like-sized fruit (about the size of a tennis ball)
- 1 cup of chopped, cooked, or canned fruit
- ½ cup of dried fruit

Low-Fat Dairy Products
- 1 cup of milk or yogurt
- 1½ to 2 ounces of cheese (about the size of a nine-volt battery)

Fish, Poultry, Lean Meats, or Eggs
- 1 ounce of cooked fish, poultry, or lean meat for a *serving* (2 to 3 ounces [about the size of a deck of cards] for a *portion*)
- 1 egg equals 1 ounce of meat

Nuts, Seeds, Legumes
- ¼ cup of cooked dry beans or peas (equivalent to 1 ounce of meat)
- ¼ cup of tofu (equivalent to 1 ounce of meat)
- 1 tablespoon of peanut or other nut butters (equivalent to 1 ounce of meat)
- ½ ounce of nuts or seeds (equivalent to 1 ounce of meat)

Plant Oils
- 1 teaspoon of plant oils
- 1 teaspoon of nuts or seeds

To be able to estimate these servings, it would be helpful to review the size of household measures, so get out the measuring cups and spoons. Estimate what ½ cup of cooked cereal would look like. That way, when eating that big bowl of oatmeal, you know that it is really two or three servings. In general, no one portion of food should be bigger than a deck of cards or a tennis ball.

THE PYRAMIDS, AGAIN

Again, information about the 2005 USDA food guide pyramid and serving size estimates can be found at *www.mypyramid.gov;* other food pyramids are available at *www.oldwayspt.org.* While none of these pyramids exactly reflects the proportion of whole natural foods our body needs to function properly, the recommendations can all be used to help point us toward healthier eating.

When our plate mirrors the recommendations from most of these pyramids and the proportions of whole natural foods our body needs, three-fourths of it should be filled with colorful high-fiber grains, fruits, and vegetables. Animal sources like lean meat, fish, poultry, or dairy should cover one-third or less. In other words, Americans need to think of animal products as a side dish or condiment, **not the focus of the meal.**

In restaurants, because of the large portions, it's a good idea to share an entrée or ask for half of the entrée to be put in a take-out box before it is served. Ask for lunch-sized portions of entrees when possible. Order an appetizer as an entrée. At home, use smaller plates, bowls, and glasses. Commit serving sizes and corresponding portion sizes to memory and eat accordingly.

Moderation is the key, with nutritional value and taste as motivation and inspiration.

Enjoying the abundance of God's gracious bounty to us should be a given, but we have the responsibility of choosing and eating foods wisely. We should be able to *"put on the full armor of God"* over a healthy body—the earthly *"temple of the living God"*! (See Ephesians 6:11 and 2 Corinthians 6:16.)

REMEMBER!

Serving size common sense should be practiced:

- Check out serving sizes on *www.mypyramid.gov.*
- Learn to estimate correct serving and portion sizes.
- Three-fourths of a plate of food should be high-fiber, colorful, complex carbohydrates.

- Use smaller plates, bowls, and glasses at home.
- Make use of the to-go box when dining out.
- Eat slowly and savor the flavor of each bite.
- During each meal, stop eating way before you start hurting!
- Moderation is the key to portion sizes.
- No one portion of any food should be bigger than a deck of cards or a tennis ball!

Remember: Gluttony is a sin!

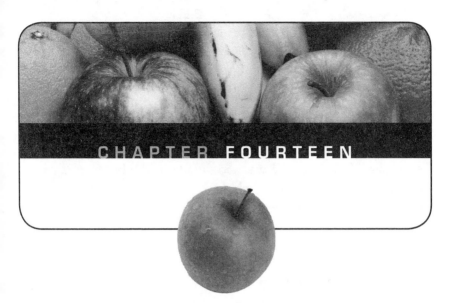

CHAPTER FOURTEEN

SEPARATING THE FRUITS FROM THE NUTS

---•---

*"Fruit trees of all kinds will grow on both banks of the river....
Every month they will bear, because the water from the sanctuary flows to them.
Their fruit will serve for food and their leaves for healing."*
—Ezekiel 47:12

*"To him who overcomes, I will give the right to eat from the tree of life,
which is in the paradise of God."*
—Revelation 2:7

HEALTHY eating is what our bodies were made for. One day when we are again in paradise with God, He will provide us exactly what we need for food as He did in the beginning. Until then, it is up to us to discern among the abundance of natural and unnatural foods available today.

LEARN TO CHOOSE

We must learn to choose what and how much we should eat for health and enjoyment. We know that for maximum nutrition, the closer a food is to the way God made it, the better it is for our bodies. So even though whole, organic, free-range, locally produced foods are the ideal, realistically we sometimes have to settle for less. We need to read labels and avoid as much of the unnatural as possible.

TAKE SUPPLEMENTS IF NEEDED

If a person is not getting enough calories daily for optimal nutrition, the doctor or dietitian may recommend supplementation of certain nutrients in the daily diet. Taking single supplements of most nutrients is not a good idea unless done under a doctor's care. Overdosing on single nutrients can cause other nutrients to become out of balance in the body. Your doctor will let you know if single supplements like calcium or iron are necessary for you. However, for most people, taking a multiple vitamin and mineral supplement daily is not a bad idea (just in case). For babies and children, the pediatrician usually recommends specific vitamin and mineral supplements at certain ages.

CONSIDER THE SOURCE

The body of knowledge from nutrition research grows so fast daily that we must all—dietitians, nurses, doctors, pharmacists, moms, dads, Jane Does, and John Does—find reliable information resources to count on. One of the best resources is the American Dietetic Association, available at *www.eatright.org* or by calling 1-800-877-1600.

Dietitians in the United States are credentialed as registered dietitians (RDs) by the profession's accrediting body, the Commission on Dietetic Registration (CDR) of the American Dietetic Association (ADA).

Always ask these questions when reading articles about nutrition and health in newspapers, magazines, journals, or books or on the Internet:

- Who is the author? Sometimes it helps to perform a Web search for the author's name.
- What are his or her credentials?
- Is a credible sponsoring institution identified?
- Is the site or article promoting or selling a particular product?
- Is the information based on scientific research or opinion?
- Is a date listed? How current is the information?
- In regard to Internet sites, are there links to other sources of information? Are the facts documented with sound scientific references, or is the information based solely on personal testimonials?
- Does the tone of the writing indicate a balanced approach?

These resources may help in evaluating Web sites:

- "The Good, The Bad & The Ugly: Or, Why It's a Good Idea to Evaluate Web Sources," available at: *http://lib.nmsu.edu/ instruction/eval.html*. From New Mexico State University, this guide includes links to examples of both good and bad Web sites.
- "Critically Analyzing Information Sources," available at Cornell University Library Web site: *http://www.library.cornell .edu/olinuris/ref/research/skill26.htm*. This quick guide helps a reader determine the relevance and authority of a resource. The next site is a useful companion guide to this resource.
- "Distinguishing Scholarly Journals from Other Periodicals," also available at Cornell University Library Web site: *http:// www.library.cornell.edu/olinuris/ref/research/skill20.html*.
- "Evaluating Information Found on the Internet," available at Johns Hopkins University, The Sheridan Libraries Web site: *http://www.library.jhu.edu/researchhelp/general/evaluating/*. This is a thoughtful guide to evaluating Web and other Internet resources for scholarly purposes.

- "Evaluation of Information Sources," available at: *http:// www.vuw.ac.nz/staff/alastair_smith/evaln/evaln.htm*. This is an extensive list of links to the many other sites available on evaluating information.

REMEMBER!

For healthy eating, choose the following:

- Whole, unprocessed foods
- 100% whole grains and cereals
- Natural unrefined plant oils and **no trans fats**
- Organic meats and dairy products
- Locally grown fruits and vegetables when possible
- Water or noncaloric beverages when thirsty
- Breakfast to start the day
- Healthy snacks and desserts
- Nutrient-dense foods, or power foods, daily
- Moderate portions (no bigger than a deck of cards or tennis ball)
- Daily multivitamin (for most people)

Remember: All natural foods are good foods...when eaten in moderation.

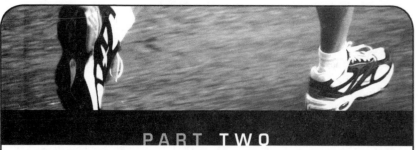

PART TWO

PHYSICAL ACTIVITY

"Six days you shall labor and do all your work."
—Deuteronomy 5:13

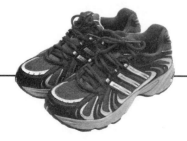

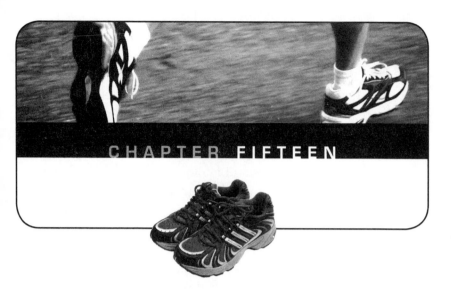

CHAPTER FIFTEEN

FEARFULLY AND WONDERFULLY MADE

———————•———————

O LORD, you have searched me and you know me....
For you created my inmost being;...
I praise you because I am fearfully and wonderfully made.
—Psalm 139 excerpts (bold added)

WHEN God created our bodies, He also provided all the food needed to fuel those bodies. In the beginning, Adam and Eve ate of the abundance of food available in the garden that God had provided—nuts, seeds, legumes, fruits, roots, and vegetables—mostly complex carbohydrates, moderate protein, and fat. After the flood, He gave humanity permission through Noah to also eat meat (Genesis 9:3). By that time, man was working hard (by the sweat of his brow!) to wrestle his food from a fallen world. With the cultivation of crops and domestication of animals, life was hard.

From this time on, until the Industrial Revolution and modern age, humans worked as their bodies were designed to—in constant daily physical activity. They ate seasonally, since there was no other choice. Frequently there was nothing to eat at all. To get through hard winters and famines, the human body has a natural mechanism of storing energy in fat cells. Our fat-storage mechanism worked beautifully until about 100 years ago. Then as technology began to take the place of physical activity, our beautifully and wonderfully made bodies began to work against us!

The body's preferred energy source has always been and will forever be the sugar glucose, which is found in carbohydrates. The carbohydrates are the main nutrients that fuel exercise of a moderate to high intensity, while fat can fuel low-intensity exercise for long periods. Proteins are generally spared to maintain and repair body tissues; they are not normally used to fuel muscle activity.

THE BODY NEEDS ACTIVITY

The US Surgeon General, the Centers for Disease Control and Prevention, and the American College of Sports Medicine all recommend that adults get a minimum of 30 minutes of moderate physical activity most days of the week, if not daily, to maintain health. Adults need 60 minutes of moderate physical activity to maintain weight and 60 to 90 minutes a day to lose weight or maintain weight loss. Children and teenagers need a minimum of 60 minutes of moderate physical activity a day. The more activity and the more intense it is, the more physical benefit the body gets, especially if that body needs to lose weight for health reasons. Physical activity may be done all at once or broken up into 10- or 15-minute periods. Moderate-intensity physical activity or exercise causes a slight but noticeable increase in breathing and heart rate. One way to gauge moderate activity is with the "talk test"—exercising hard enough to break a sweat but not so hard you can't comfortably carry on a conversation. The USDA gives examples of different levels of exercise:

Moderate Physical Activity

- Walking briskly (about 3½ miles per hour) as though you were late to a meeting
- Hiking
- Gardening/yard work
- Dancing
- Golf (walking and carrying clubs)
- Bicycling (less than 10 miles per hour)
- Weight training (general light workout)

Moderate-intensity activities are those that are fast enough or strenuous enough to burn three to six times as much energy per minute as sitting quietly. Exercising longer, harder, or both can bring even greater health benefits.

Vigorous Physical Activity

- Running/jogging (5 miles per hour)
- Bicycling (more than 10 miles per hour)
- Swimming (freestyle laps)
- Aerobics
- Walking very fast (4½ miles per hour)
- Heavy yard work (chopping wood, for example)
- Weight lifting (vigorous effort)
- Basketball (competitive)

Moderate or vigorous activity should be in addition to everyday activities, although routine activities like vacuuming, mopping, raking leaves, washing the car, or walking up steps add to overall activity. When most people were still physically active just living their everyday lives, metabolism worked quite well, thank you. The calories that were eaten were burned up—even those evil simple sugars and saturated fats!

LEARN FROM THE AMISH

David Bassett, a professor at the University of Tennessee, has researched the physical activity and health of a community of Amish people, who still live as most people did 150 years ago. His findings were published in the *Medicine and Science in Sports and Exercise* journal (36 [2004]: 79–85). Wearing pedometers, the Amish went about their everyday activities. The men spent about 10 hours a week doing heavy work like plowing, shoeing horses, tossing hay bales, and digging. The women spent about 3½ hours a week at heavy chores. Men spent 55 hours a week in moderate activity and were taking an average of 18,000 steps a day (9 miles). Women reported 45 hours a week of moderate chores, such as gardening and doing laundry, and were taking an average of 14,000 steps a day (7 miles). Their reported diet is similar to the pre-World War II diet in the US, with lots of meat, potatoes, gravy, and, yes, even pies and cakes. They ate a substantial breakfast, their main meal at noon, and a substantial dinner, too. This research showed that the Amish men ate about 3,600 calories a day; the women, around 2,100 calories. Bassett commented, "It really struck me that we have come a long way from our biological heritage to what we do today. The amount of physical activity required to live in today's society is very low."

No kidding! In other words, our way of modern eating and inactive living is not compatible with our genes. If we want that pie, we have to work it off or walk it off! For metabolism, the simple formula is calories in equal calories out for maintenance of weight. A greater number of calories in than out means weight gain, and taking in fewer calories than are worked off means weight loss. Of course, in reality, it is much more complex, but as far as the body's metabolism interprets the equation, that is the bottom line.

STRESS MAKES A DIFFERENCE

Stress is and always has been a normal response of the body and mind. Life events like marriage, divorce, births, deaths, disappointments, starting or ending school or jobs, arguments, finances, deadlines, or traffic jams are all normal stressors. Social isolation and loneliness, job insecurity, peer pressure, broken families, hurriedness, and technology are just the tip of the iceberg of our daily stress load.

Stress-induced hormones (mainly cortisol) from chronic stress can affect our health by raising the risks of heart disease, stroke, diabetes, cancer, gastrointestinal problems, eating disorders, depression, sleep disorders, fatigue, and memory loss, among other conditions. Extreme sudden emotional stress, like news of a death, can actually cause a heart attack. Researchers have now shown that stress also weakens the immune system. This has implications for increasing risk for many other diseases ranging from the common cold and flu to rheumatoid arthritis and Crohn's disease. Prevention of stress-related diseases must obviously include ways to relieve and decrease stress. This includes eating healthy foods that encourage the excretion of the antistress hormones serotonin, endorphins, and dopamine and eating enough mixed meals (carbohydrate, protein, and fat) during the day to keep glucose levels constant. But stress can also be reduced by means other than diet; let's look at physical activity, for one.

ACTIVITY LOWERS STRESS

In addition to eating healthy foods and keeping the blood glucose levels normal and constant, appropriate physical activity lowers stress levels in the body—as do maintaining normal body weight for height, prayer, meditation, relaxation, and sleep, also. Lowering stress levels, in turn, lowers risks for heart disease, stroke, diabetes, cancer, osteoporosis, dementia, and depression. Physical activity improves intellectual capacity, increases productivity, strengthens the immune system, strengthens the skeletal system, helps prevent chronic back pain, improves digestive system function, improves sleep, increases resting metabolic rate, and increases personal energy.

Does physical activity really do all that? Absolutely! Our bodies were made for activity! In this book, we are going to look at ways to incorporate activity into our daily lives, focusing on activities that build **strength, endurance, and flexibility—the three components of fitness.** Membership at a gym or health club is not necessary in order to be physically fit. The activity of daily living (household chores and daily routines) provide some exercise; that in combination with additional intentional activities of extra steps, different modes of exercise, sports, and stretching can improve emotional, spiritual, and physical health.

THE BODY HAS RHYTHMS

In recent years, one of the most amazing discoveries about the body has been that it has cycles and rhythms like much of nature. In fact, some of the rhythms of body and mind are tied to nature. When functioning properly, the human circadian rhythm—or internal body clock of a 24-hour cycle of light and dark, wakefulness and sleep—responds to morning light and the darkening of evening and night. This circadian rhythm sets most other bodily processes. At regular intervals each day, the body tends to become hungry, tired, active, listless, energized. Body temperature, blood pressure, hormone levels, and urine flow rise and fall in this relatively predictable, rhythmic pattern that is under the control of exposure to sunlight and darkness.

Weekly rhythms of seven days, called circaseptan rhythms, are also now recognized. These rhythms are related to the immune system, blood pressure, heartbeat, and stress hormones. All living things—plants, animals, insects, and even single cells—seem to have this seven-day rhythm. Should it be surprising that scientists have determined that these rhythms are inborn in nature? God created 24-hour periods called days, and seven of those days are a week. A lunar month has about four seven-day cycles. God's created order continues in our bodies just as in all of nature.

Is this a coincidence? I think not. The significance of the number seven in the Bible is not to be ignored. The number seven is used as a symbol for completion and rest in the Creation. The number seven indicates the fullness of God's revelation and

God's oath or promise. The Bible begins with the seven days of the Creation and ends with the seven seals of revelation. Now science is showing us that this number of completion is woven into all of life. God is the "*Alpha and Omega, the beginning and the ending*" (Revelation 1:8 KJV). It should be no surprise that the central feature of our biological time clock is that the components themselves reflect God's creation.

> *For by him all things were created: things in heaven and on earth, visible and invisible, whether thrones or powers or rulers or authorities; all things were created by him and for him. He is before all things, and in him all things hold together.*
> —Colossians 1:16–17

Stop and think about the marvelous gift of your body. Saint Augustine said, "People travel to wonder at the height of the mountains, at the huge waves of the sea, at the long courses of rivers, at the vast compass of the ocean, at the circular motion of the stars, and yet they pass by themselves without wondering." How sad. Man, as meant to be, is the temple of the Holy Spirit. Every Christian is the priest of that temple. We have the responsibility to take care of it by the Creator's Handbook.

Regular meals from **whole natural foods**, daily **moderate physical activity,** and **appropriate rest** work with metabolism, not against it. Healthy living begins and ends at the cellular level. This is how God made us and the design hasn't changed.

REMEMBER!

We were created with a purpose; we are *"fearfully and wonderfully made"* **(Psalm 139:14).**

- God made our bodies to be physically active and provided whole foods for fuel.

- The stresses and increased inactivity of modern life and the convenience of processed foods that come with that same modern life throw off metabolism and natural energy balance.

- Reducing life and body stresses, increasing physical activity in our everyday life, and choosing whole natural foods are worth the effort they require.

Remember: The body's metabolism, which is regulated by rest, uses whole natural foods to fuel physical activity.

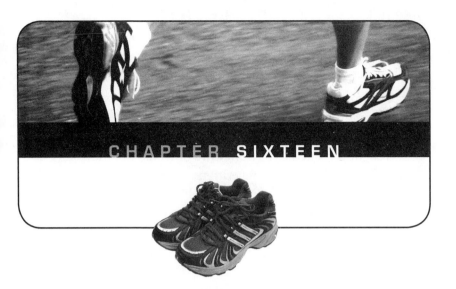

CHAPTER SIXTEEN

THE SWEAT OF YOUR BROW

•

*By the sweat of your brow you will eat your food until you return to the ground,
since from it you were taken.*
—Genesis 3:19

*Then Miriam the prophetess, Aaron's sister, took a tambourine in her hand,
and all the women followed her, with tambourines and dancing.*
—Exodus 15:20

OUR body was made for physical activity. It makes our metabolism happy! A happy metabolism burns energy and lets our body systems know that all is well. We eat and burn that food energy for metabolism, digestion, and the activity of our body's 600 muscles. We rest and the body repairs those muscles and organs for the next day of activity.

PHYSICAL FITNESS

Physical activity or work incorporates all three components of fitness: strength, endurance, and flexibility. Combined intentional activities, such as walking, jogging, or resistance exercises, should incorporate all three.

- **Strength** is related to a strong core or trunk and the ability of muscles to lift and make repetitions.
- **Endurance** is usually defined as aerobic endurance and refers to the ability of the body to provide oxygen to the muscles during sustained activity.
- **Flexibility** is the range of joints related to stretching.

Physical fitness includes all of these areas as well as body composition. Body composition can tell us how physically fit we are since it is the ratio of fat to muscle mass in our bodies. Athletes or fit individuals with defined muscles often have more muscle than fat. Muscle weighs more that fat, so those persons could possibly be considered overweight or obese according to a height-to-weight ratio or even a body mass index (BMI) chart. A really skinny model could actually be too fat inside if she has little muscle, but the height-to-weight ratio or BMI would label her underweight. Waist size related to tallness (waist-to-tallness ratio—WTR) is probably a better indicator of body composition and risk for disease related to obesity than is height-to-weight ratio or BMI.

Since abdominal fat puts a person at risk for obesity-related disease, waist circumference should be kept down to 38 inches or less for a man. For a 5-foot-5-inch-tall woman, the waist measurement guideline is 34 inches or less. To determine the upper limit of a healthy waistline (in inches) according to a specific height, multiply height in inches by 0.55 for men and 0.53 for women. That gives a fairly good idea. The Web site for the originator of the WTR, Dr. Margaret Ashwell, is available at *www.ashwell.uk.com*.

WHAT IS A HEALTHY BODY?

We do **not** have to look like our favorite athletes or models to have a healthy body. Healthy bodies come in many shapes and sizes. About one-fourth of US adults are sedentary and another third are not active enough to reach a healthy level of fitness. For admitted sedentary people—and there are plenty of them—just a little daily activity can reduce risk of most of the diseases related to obesity. The National Heart, Lung, and Blood Institute, the Cooper Institute, and the National Institutes of Health have shown that small changes in lifestyle that increase moderate-intensity activities lower risk of heart disease, stroke, and type 2 diabetes.

Increasing activity may be as simple as taking more steps during the day: taking longer walks on the way to office meetings, walking around airports instead of sitting while waiting for a plane, walking around the soccer field during a child's practices and games, and walking more with friends and family during or after work. The Cooper Institute of Aerobics Research advises that approximately 10,000 is the number of steps needed each day to meet the established guidelines for physical activity set by the American College of Sports Medicine and the Centers for Disease Control and Prevention. This number of steps each day may be helpful in lowering body fat, improving blood pressure, and increasing cardiorespiratory (aerobic) fitness.

The standard of 10,000 steps was originally started in Japan almost 40 years ago. Walking 10,000 steps is the equivalent of going about 5 miles. The 10,000 steps goal puts the focus on the accumulation of activity across the whole day as we go about our routines. In a normal day—just living and working—most people take about 3,000 steps. Unfortunately, some people don't even take 1,000! Walking one block is equivalent to taking about 200 steps, and one mile, about 2,000. Most of us would have to do some intentional walking throughout the day to end up with 10,000. Remember, the activity can be accumulated in ten-minute increments, and ten minutes of walking is about 1,200 steps! If you are sedentary (taking fewer than 3,000 steps a day), increase daily steps gradually—by

500 each week. Using a pedometer, calculate how many steps you take in a day. For the first week, aim at walking 500 more steps a day. The next week, aim at 1,000 more a day. Keep increasing by 500 until you are taking 10,000 steps daily. Steps matter!

Check out these related resources:

- *www.justmove.org*
- *www.shapeup.org*
- *www.thewalkingsite.com* (offers a beginner's walking schedule)
- *Great Shape: The First Fitness Guide for Large Women* by Pat Lyons and Debby Burgard

THE DAILY GRIND

Work: mop, sweep, vacuum, mow the lawn, wash the car, trim the hedges, carry the groceries, put away the groceries, pull weeds, make the bed, scrub the tub, scrub the toilet, and fold the laundry.

Oh, come on—I don't like it either, but we all have to do it. At least it isn't as hard as it used to be, according to Garrison Keillor ("The Old Scout: Ambition and the Honesty of Everyday Work," A Prairie Home Companion), who himself has been told he works too hard. He stirs our memories as he describes the way his mother worked, sometimes with the help of her six children. Her list of usual chores included cleaning, cooking, washing clothes, and hanging them on the line, but one particular chore has etched a vivid memory for Keillor. His description of the "late-summer orgy of canning" takes those of us who have been there back in time. The children picked every last tomato, string bean, ear of corn, and cucumber and then helped chop and slice the vegetables. The kitchen was a literal boiler room, with clouds of steam spewing from the pressure cooker and teakettles. His mother, with hair as wet as if she had been swimming, slaved away, washing jars, steaming tomatoes, and canning.

See what I mean? Now, that was work! But even these days, with our many modern conveniences, everyday activities can still burn off many calories.

According to researchers at the Centers for Disease Control and Prevention as well as the US Surgeon General, household tasks, such as pushing a vacuum, folding clean clothes, and scrubbing the toilet, qualify as moderate physical exercise. **Housework utilizes all of the body's muscle groups, which builds strength, endurance, and flexibility.** For example, picking up the children's toys works the arm and shoulder muscles. Hauling those toys throughout the house and up the stairs works the legs and buttocks. Walking the length of the house while vacuuming provides a full body workout that also burns calories and increases heart rate—if done **fast.**

Many experts agree that any household chore can become aerobic if a person strives to reach the target heart rate zone. (To estimate your target rate, subtract your age from 220—this provides your maximum heart rate; 50% to 90% of this number is the target heart rate zone.) To make a chore more aerobic, push to work faster and scrub harder and longer. Lower-intensity chores include doing laundry, making the beds, ironing, washing dishes, and cooking. For housework that provides moderate intensity, sweep the kitchen or sidewalk, wash windows or walls, and mop. High-intensity chores involve moving furniture or boxes and carrying heavier items up and down the stairs.

When using daily cleaning activities as a way to greater fitness and strength, it's important to remember to bend properly, using the legs rather than back. Start daily household chores with slow, gentle stretches. When stretching, it is always better to ease into them, and if the stretch hurts, go slower until the muscle feels warm. Another good tip to remember is to alternate cleaning activities to prevent overworking particular muscle groups and to avoid burnout. For instance, vacuum a couple of rooms, then scrub the bathroom, do some laundry, or make the beds.

Finally, in order to get a good workout, you must be moderately active at least 30 minutes every day—10 minutes at a time. If you've been sedentary up to this point, start slowly with 10 minutes of moderate activity and work up. Pay attention to how you feel as you perform each task. If you begin to feel too tired or short of breath, slow down or move to an easier chore.

Let's just see how many calories we can burn by doing common chores for 30 minutes:

- Vacuuming: between 75 and 125 calories, depending on how fast we do it
- Making beds: 70 calories
- Cooking: 40 to 50 calories
- Raking leaves: 110 calories
- Lawn mowing: between 150 and 225 calories, depending on how much we have to push

So—get those mops and brooms out and attack those floors. Be vigorous about dusting! If you want even more action than the chores provide, just go up and down stairs a couple of times between cleaning or loads of laundry. The American Council on Exercise (*www.acefitness.org*) states that walking stairs can burn as many calories in a 30-minute period as jogging at a 12-minute mile pace or cycling at 12 to 14 miles per hour. That translates to burning over 300 calories for a normal-weight man or woman. Plus, the faster you go, the more calories are burned. And the activity can be broken down into 10-minute intervals, making it even more doable!

WALKING, JOGGING, KICKBOXING, DANCING—JUST NAME IT

For most Americans who don't have active jobs—we are not all mail carriers or lumberjacks—intentional activity is needed in addition to everyday activities. Workout videos, dance videos, and exercise machines are endless in number but may be limited as to when and where they can be used. The one intentional activity that most of us can do almost anytime or anywhere is walk. If you must walk inside because it is too cold or too hot outside or for safety reasons, the AARP gives several tips at their Web site (*www.aarp.org*). Consider these suggestions:

- **Shopping malls.** Malls often open early just so people can walk. Check the local mall for walking hours. There may even be a mall walking club you can join.

- **Schools.** Many schools let community members use the gymnasium during off-hours. Also college and universities typically have indoor tracks and gymnasiums that are open to the public during certain hours.
- **Museums.** Enjoy some culture while walking through all the long halls in a museum. This is especially nice for leisurely walks.
- **Convention centers.** These are large spaces open to the public. Just check first to see if an event is going on.
- **Airports, train stations.** Many airports and train stations have long halls to walk through and are open to the public every day of the week.
- **Warehouse stores.** Walk up and down the aisles of these hardware, discount, or supercenter stores. Consider leaving your cash behind so you can focus on walking, not shopping! Or if you must shop—walk all the aisles before choosing your items.
- **The office.** If you work in a large office, take the stairs to a restroom on a different floor during the day. A few trips to the restroom at the other end of the office can help the steps add up quicker.
- **Your home.** Even if you don't have a treadmill, you can clear off the floors to walk around rooms in your house, basement, or even garage. And don't forget the stairs!

Walking could turn into jogging. Just think of that! If your knees can take it, jogging picks up the workout! To begin, just increase the walking pace. Remember, the longer and more intense the activity, the more fat will be burned. Walking or jogging can be alternated with any other moderate activity just to keep it fun. There are zillions of workout videos on the market, ranging from kickboxing to belly dancing and everything between. A good Web site that gives reviews is *www.justaboutfitness.com*.

In order to increase lean body mass, which is required for burning more calories, strength training can be alternated with aerobic activity. Remember also that aerobic activity and deep breathing help increase the lungs' capacity to deliver more oxygen to tissues for burning energy. Increased oxygen + more muscle mass = burning more calories, even at rest!

SHOW ME THE MUSCLE

Scientific research has shown that physical activity can slow the physiological consequences of aging. While aerobic exercise, such as walking, jogging, or swimming, has many excellent health benefits (maintains the heart and lungs and increases cardiovascular fitness and endurance), it does not make muscles strong. Strength or resistance training does. Studies have shown that lifting weights or using resistance training two or three times a week increases strength by building lean muscle mass and bone density. Functional strength training builds core strength, balance, and coordination for general fitness and improves the ability to perform everyday activities.

In midlife, adults begin to lose muscle mass as they age. Indeed, if you don't use it, you lose it! Individuals who have more muscle mass have a higher metabolic rate and more mitochondria (energy factories for the cells) in their muscles. Muscle is active tissue that consumes and burns calories, while stored fat uses very little energy. Strength training can provide up to a 15% increase in metabolic rate, which is enormously helpful for weight loss and long-term weight control.

Strength training in the elderly has been shown to increase muscle and bone mass, muscle strength, flexibility, balance, self-confidence, and self-esteem. Strength training also helps reduce the symptoms of various chronic diseases, such as arthritis, depression, type 2 diabetes, osteoporosis, sleep disorders, and heart disease, and when combined with balance training, can reduce falls. New guidelines from the American College of Sports Medicine suggest strength training two or three times a week. Be sure to give your muscles at least one day of rest between workouts. Two sessions per week is suggested, because that number gives you the training benefits and is also quite manageable from a time perspective. For core strengthening, start your weight or resistance workouts with abdominal exercises. To strengthen abs daily, every time you think about it, sit up or stand up straight and contract the abdominal muscles. Eventually this will become a habit. For your overall workout program, consider alternating aerobic exercise like walking, jogging, or dancing with strength training. Always consult your physician before starting any exercise program, of course.

Web sites, videos, and books for weight and resistance training are abundant. To start, check out these:

- *www.bellaonline.com*
- *www.pilates.com*
- *www.workoutsforyou.com*
- *www.workoutsforwomen.com*
- *http://weboflife.nasa.gov/exerciseandaging/toc.html*
- *Strength Training for Seniors* by Wayne Westcott
- *Functional Fitness for Older Adults* by Patricia Brill
- *Functional Fitness* by Larkin Barnett
- *The Pilates Body* by Brooke Siler
- *Essentials of Strength Training and Conditioning* by Thomas Baechle, Roger Earle, and the National Strength and Conditioning Association
- "Weight Lifting for Absolute Beginners" by Jonni and Jessie Good, a great downloadable strength program available at: *http://www.weight-lifting-exercise.com/?hop=fatburn*

It is always a good idea to get a hands-on demonstration of exercises from a fitness instructor before beginning. Once you have the know-how, you may want to set up a home gym for the sake of convenience. The following lists provide ideas for exercising at home with varying levels of limited funds:

No Budget
- Use soup cans as weights for upper-body training.
- Work out with television exercise classes.

- Borrow exercise videos and fitness magazines from the library.
- Do the exercises that do not require equipment: stretches, jumping jacks, squats, lunges, triceps dips, abduction and adduction lifts, heel raises, back extension, abdominal crunches, push-ups, and push-offs. And remember, stair climbing is always free!

Low Budget
- Purchase a set of resistance bands for strength training.
- Rent videotapes from the video store.
- Purchase a step for cardiovascular workouts.
- Buy a jump rope.
- Get a mat for abdominal work and stretches.

Medium Budget
- Purchase a set of free weights.
- Buy an assortment of physical activity videotapes.
- Get a mat.
- Buy one piece of top-quality cardio equipment (such as a tread-mill, stationary bicycle, stair-climber, ski machine, rower, or cross trainer). Be sure to purchase equipment that is sturdy, has safety features (especially if you have small children), and is something you enjoy using.

In summary, reasons to include resistance strength training in a workout routine are abundant:

- **To build muscle strength.** Adults lose between five and seven pounds of muscle every decade after age 20. Strength training prevents muscle loss.
- **To improve functional strength and flexibility.** This is impor-tant because it can help keep you safe during daily activities and make you less vulnerable to falls or other injuries.
- **To increase bone mass and density.** Weight-bearing and resis-tance exercises can help protect against osteoporosis, a disease in which bones become fragile and more likely to break.

- To lower body fat—especially abdominal fat!
- To reduce resting blood pressure.
- To reduce low back pain.
- To reduce the pain of osteoarthritis and rheumatoid arthritis.
- **To reduce symptoms of other chronic diseases.** Strength training can help to reduce the symptoms of depression, heart disease, type 2 diabetes, osteoporosis, and sleep disorders.
- **To enhance personal appearance.** Improving strength and physique can also be a plus for self-confidence and self-esteem.
- **To improve your golf game.** Believe it or not, strength training can improve golf performance by increasing club head speed and driving power. It can also help enhance other physical activities, such as tennis and cycling.

IMPORTANCE OF THE WARM-UP AND STRETCH

A warm muscle is much more easily stretched than a cold muscle. Never stretch a cold muscle. Always warm up first to get blood circulating throughout the body and into the muscles. A warm-up should be a slow, rhythmic exercise of larger muscle groups and is done before an activity. Riding a bicycle or walking works well. This provides the body with a period of adjustment between rest and the activity. The warm-up should last about 5 to 10 minutes and should be similar to the activity that you are about to do, but at a much lower intensity.

Once you have warmed up at a low intensity for about 5 to 10 minutes and have gotten the muscles warm, then stretch. Benefits of stretching are numerous; let's consider a few:

- **Increased flexibility and better range of motion of the joints.** Flexible muscles can improve daily performance. Tasks like lifting packages, bending to tie shoes, or hurrying to catch a bus become easier and less tiring. Flexibility tends to diminish with age, but it can be regained and maintained.
- **Improved circulation.** Stretching increases blood flow to muscles. Blood flowing to muscles provides nourishment and gets rid of waste by-products in the muscle tissue. Improved circulation helps shorten recovery time for any muscle injury.

- **Better posture.** Frequent stretching helps keep muscles from getting tight, allowing proper posture to be maintained. Good posture can minimize discomfort and keep aches and pains at a minimum.
- **Stress relief.** Stretching relaxes the tight, tense muscles that often accompany stress.
- **Enhanced coordination.** Maintaining the full range of motion through joints helps maintain better balance. Coordination and balance help keep a person mobile and less prone to injury from falls.

In addition to stretching major muscle groups before exercise, stretch muscles and joints that are routinely used at work or play. Sport-specific stretching prepares muscles for a particular sport or activity. For example, if you frequently play tennis or golf, doing a few extra shoulder stretches loosens the muscles around the shoulder joints, making them feel less tight and more ready for action. Use active isolated stretching that works one muscle at a time.

Resources for warm-up and stretching routines can be found at the Web sites and in the books mentioned previously for exercise. Also, check these out:

- *www.thestretchinghandbook.com*
- *Office Yoga: 75 Simple Stretches for Busy People* by Darrin Zeer
- *Stretching in the Office* by Bob Anderson

For simple stretching and deep breathing at a desk or workstation (see chapter 19 for deep-breathing techniques), try the following:

- Sit straight up in the chair or stand.

  Stretch arms over your head, interlock fingers, and turn palms toward the ceiling.

  Breathe in deeply, and while exhaling, stretch arms and torso to the right.

  Breathe in deeply again, and while exhaling, return to the middle.

Breathe in deeply, exhale, and stretch to the left.

Breathe in deeply again, and on the exhale, return to the middle.

• As you breathe in deeply, lift shoulders toward your ears.

Exhale and let them fall.

Repeat three times.

• Sit on chair with your feet placed flat on the floor in front of you.

On an exhale, twist to the right, placing your right hand on the back of the chair and your left hand on the side of the chair. Hold for a few seconds.

Return to the middle.

Switch hands and directions.

• Pull out a desk drawer and prop your foot on it while breathing in deeply.

Breathe slowly out and lean over that leg.

Breathe in again and hold for 20 to 30 seconds.

Exhale slowly.

A fitness ball can also be used to start stretching at work. Sit on the ball and roll forward until the ball is under the lower back. Gradually lean shoulders and head backwards over the ball. Stay in this position for 20 to 30 seconds and repeat. Don't let your neck bend too far backward. Repeat this exercise several times a day. It stretches the back and can help relieve tension headache and stress. Stretching helps combat the aches and pains of sitting at a desk or keyboard all day.

Some great office exercises with illustrations can be found at *http://exercise.about.com/cs/exerciseworkouts/l/blofficeworkout.htm.*

GOLF OR TENNIS, ANYONE?

Who said that leisure sports are not a workout? Well, staying in the golf cart might make that true. However, if you've ever walked a golf course carrying or pulling your bag, you **know** that it's definitely a workout, but lots of fun. The United States Golf Association (USGA) is encouraging golfers to ditch their carts and take up their bags and walk! Studies have shown that the strong health benefits of walking can also help protect golfers against heart disease. According to *Golf Science International*, four hours of playing golf by foot—*walking* the course—is comparable to a 45-minute fitness class! That's good news, since golf is unique in the way it can motivate middle-aged and elderly individuals to walk a fairly long distance on a regular basis.

A Hawaiian study showed that men who walk 1½ miles or more each day have less than half the rate of heart problems compared with those who walk less than a quarter mile. Most importantly, the results showed that it doesn't matter what the walking speed is, as long as the distance is covered. One great positive that comes from the use of the motorized golf bag carriers that are becoming more popular is the benefit of walking. In fact, a group of golfers started using these carriers 30 years ago in their sixties; they are now still walking the course in their nineties! That's great! So if golf is your game—get out there for health benefits and a great time with your friends and family and *walk* the course. Go to *www.walkinggolf.com* for more information and inspiration.

Another favorite American leisure sport is tennis. Playing tennis on a regular basis is excellent exercise. Playing tennis at a moderate to vigorous intensity on a regular basis is a good way to get aerobic exercise. Muscles are exercised and calories are burned. Studies have shown that singles tennis burns more calories than does the doubles game, of course, but even doubles can give the exercise benefits of light weight lifting or bowling.

To kick tennis up a notch, try Cardio Tennis; it's a new, fun group activity featuring drills to give players of all abilities an ultimate, high-energy workout. Taught by a teaching professional, Cardio Tennis includes warm-up, cardio-workout, and cool-down phases. If you are looking for a new way to get in shape and to burn calories, Cardio Tennis may be for you. There are local programs in most every state. To learn more, go to *www.cardiotennis.com*.

Other leisure sports that are great physical activities and family fun include volleyball, skating, cycling, mountain biking, climbing, surfing, winter sports, and many more. Pass on your passions to your family. Teach your children the fundamentals and include them in your sport. Some of my best memories are of playing golf as a child with my patient mother. The best part was getting my peanut butter crackers and Mountain Dew (sorry) between the ninth and tenth holes! We had fun, no matter how many balls I lost in the woods and in the water. Pass on the fun!

REMEMBER!

If we don't use it, we lose it!

- Our bodies were made for physical activity.
- The three components of fitness are strength, endurance, and flexibility.
- Approximately 10,000 is the number of steps needed each day.
- Housework utilizes all of the body's muscle groups and can build strength, endurance, and flexibility.
- Strength training can provide up to a 15% increase in metabolic rate, which is enormously helpful for weight loss and long-term weight control.
- Always warm up and stretch before exercise.
- Performing stretching exercises at work helps combat the aches and pains of sitting at a desk or keyboard all day.
- Leisure sports, too, can provide a good workout.

Remember: The sweat means you are really working your body, and that's good!

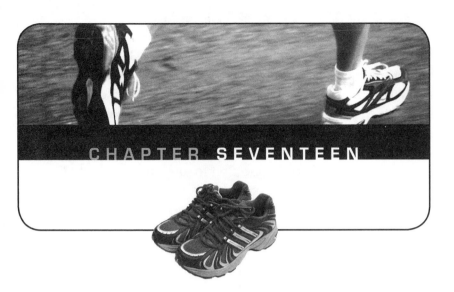

CHAPTER SEVENTEEN

JUST GET MOVING

———————•———————

The LORD said to Abram… "Go, walk through the length and breadth of the land, for I am giving it to you."
—Genesis 13:14, 17

Then the LORD said to Joshua,… "March around the city [Jericho] once with all the armed men. Do this for six days."
—Joshua 6:2–3

DON'T you love hearing the stories about how 60 years ago, your grandparents walked two miles to school through rain, sleet, and snow and carried a tin pail with their lunch? Well, even I walked to school, and that was only 45 years ago! (Yes, I admit it.) My, times have changed!

PRIVATE TRANSPORTATION—THE DEATH OF ACTIVE LIVES

Suburban sprawl began to take off after World War II; and in the United States, suburban has become our middle name. Around the world in places where suburbs also exist, public transportation is usually available. However, in the US, where most Americans seem to have several cars in their driveways, many cities have little or no bus, rail, or subway connection to surrounding suburbs.

In 2003, Vital Signs reported that the average car in the United States is driven 10% more per year than a car in the United Kingdom, about 50% more than one in Germany, and almost 200% more than a car in Japan. I have seen people get in the car to go to their mailbox! We are not walking because we are all driving! We are driving either because we live too far from our lives or there are no sidewalks or it is not safe to walk. As we become aware of our personal inactivity on a daily basis, we must find ways to get out and just move!

It was about 50 years ago that the mall, as we know it, was born. So suburbia and the mall syndrome combined with the "mart" syndrome, as in K- and Wal-, have moved our lives farther and farther away from where we actually live. However, with high gas prices and global warming looming, we may see an interest return for more public transportation and urban or small-town living. Those concepts are already booming in some areas of the country.

WALKABLE DOWNTOWNS AND SMALL TOWNS

Downtown areas in America's large cities are being reclaimed and revitalized, and more and more old-fashioned neighborhoods and small towns are being designed and built. The first "new" small town that I experienced was Mt Laurel, near Birmingham, Alabama. Sixteen years ago, when we came back from Venezuela and I started teaching undergraduate food and nutrition classes, I found a wonderful organic farm and farmers market in Mt Laurel. I grew to appreciate the farmer and Mt Laurel as I took my food and nutrition classes on field trips there every year. In Mt Laurel, the school, churches, restaurants, florist, and city center are all connected by sidewalks, just like the small south Alabama town where I visited my grandmother every summer.

A group of urban planners, especially those known as "new urbanists," have re-embraced the quaint idea that small-town life is the best. After focusing for years on Americans' diets, health experts have turned to assess the degree to which the American car dependency contributes to obesity, hypertension, coronary disease, diabetes, asthma, and even mental disorders, like anxiety and depression. With the results showing links between suburbs and risks for these conditions, the public health fields are beginning to study the effect of urban sprawl on health and to try to find solutions. The new urbanism puts the importance of place back in the community, where the people are the most important and most valuable commodity.

Small-town living, whether in a new or revitalized community, brings a higher quality of life and better places to live, work, and play. It means less traffic congestion and **less driving.** It means a healthier lifestyle with more walking, with the close proximity to retail and service, and less stress. Pedestrian-friendly communities give residents more of an opportunity to know each other. One of the things I miss about Venezuela is knowing my baker, butcher, and vegetable and fruit vendor (who sold from his truck)! Small-town living gives the children more freedom to play and the elderly and the poor more freedom to live independently and get jobs since they do not need a car. Children can walk or bike to school. More diverse mom-and-pop shops and stores with local owners are present and involved in the community. A lot of gasoline money is saved, since fewer people have to drive and own cars. A better sense of place, community, and ownership exists.

I have said many times that I felt more at home in my little neighborhood in the enormous city of Caracas, Venezuela, than in the life we live in suburban Birmingham, where we literally drive everywhere. That is really a shame. But there is hope! Just recently in the commercial district near where we live, the city began putting in sidewalks to connect some of our schools with each other and the library! That is so exciting!

PROGRAMS PROMOTING THE ACTIVE LIFE

Planning boards and public works officials in other cities have begun getting the message and are making it easier for people to walk around. Several large metropolitan cities have budgeted millions of dollars to install sidewalks. Priorities for sidewalks will go to areas around schools. A study released by the Surface Transportation Policy Project, a research and advocacy group in Washington, found that 71% of parents with school-age children walked to school themselves as children, but only 18% of their own children walk to school.

The Partnership for a Walkable America is a national coalition working to improve the conditions for walking in America and to increase the number of Americans who walk regularly. The members are national governmental agencies and nonprofit organizations concerned about health, safety, and the environment. Visit the Web site at *www.walkableamerica.org.*

The Centers for Disease Control and Prevention (CDC) has developed a program named **KidsWalk-to-School**. This is a community-based program that aims to increase opportunities for daily physical activity by encouraging children to walk to and from school in groups accompanied by adults. At the same time, the program advocates for communities to build partnerships with the school, PTA, local police department, department of public works, civic associations, local politicians, and businesses to create an environment that is supportive of walking and bicycling to school safely. By creating active and safe routes to school, walking to school can once again be a safe, fun, and pleasant part of children's daily routine. The benefits of KidsWalk-to-School are plentiful:

- Increased levels of daily physical activity for children
- Increased likelihood that children and adults will choose to walk and bike for other short-distance trips
- Improved neighborhood safety

- Fewer cars traveling through the neighborhood
- Fewer cars congesting the pickup and drop-off points at the school
- Friendlier neighborhoods as people get out and about, interacting with one another

A **walking school bus,** an idea developed by the CDC and US Department of Transportation, is a group of children walking to school with one or more adults. If that sounds simple, it is, and that's part of the beauty of the walking school bus. It can be as informal as two families taking turns walking their children to school or as structured as a route with meeting points, a timetable, and a regularly rotated schedule of trained volunteers. A variation on the walking school bus is the **bicycle train**, in which adults supervise children riding their bikes to school. The flexibility of the walking school bus makes it appealing to communities of all sizes. The CDC recommends one adult for every six children. If children are aged four to six, one adult per three children is recommended. If children are aged ten or older, fewer adults may be needed. Walking school bus guidelines may be found at the Web site *www.walkingschoolbus.org*.

Congress approved $612 million for a new **Safe Routes to School** program as part of the federal transportation bill that was adopted in 2005. The federal legislation was designed to benefit children in primary and middle schools. Funds will be distributed over a five-year period. The purposes of the program, as stated in the bill are as follows:

- To enable and encourage children, including those with disabilities, to walk and bicycle to school
- To make bicycling and walking to school a safer and more appealing transportation alternative, thereby encouraging a healthy and active lifestyle from an early age
- To facilitate the planning, development, and implementation of projects and activities that will improve safety and reduce traffic, fuel consumption, and air pollution in the vicinity of schools

Funding will be provided to each state's department of transportation on a formula basis calculated from school enrollment. Eligible activities for funding under Safe Routes to School include both infrastructure projects and non-infrastructure-related projects, including sidewalk improvement, on-street bicycle facilities, off-street bicycle and pedestrian facilities, secure bicycle parking, and traffic diversion improvements in the vicinity of schools. The federal Safe Routes to School program has further established a National Safe Routes to School Clearinghouse to develop information and educational programs on Safe Routes to School and to provide technical assistance and disseminate techniques and strategies used for successful Safe Routes to School programs. Each state is also required to create a full-time position for a Safe Routes to School coordinator, which will establish a point person for Safe Routes to School within each department of transportation in all 50 states. Amen!

WALKING AND PUBLIC TRANSPORTATION

In order to get the rest of America walking, we must improve public transportation in both urban and rural areas. Public transportation encourages people to get out of their cars and adopt more active lifestyles. America's first subway system was opened in Boston in 1897 followed by New York in 1904 and Philadelphia in 1908. Subways continued to grow in number and usage through the first half of the twentieth century. After 1946, however, Americans turned to the automobile, and subway use decreased for the next 25 years until the early 1970s. The building of San Francisco's light rail system marked the beginning of a revival for American subways. Now many cities such as Atlanta, Miami, Baltimore, and Washington DC have similar systems.

The Web site *www.lightrailnow.org* gives information about light rail systems all over the world. As gas and oil prices soar worldwide, the pressure for expansion of light rail systems is expected to increase. More information about public transportation in the US in both urban and rural areas can be found at the following Web sites:

- American Public Transportation Association,
  www.publictransportation.org
- The Community Transportation Association of America,
  www.ctaa.org
- The National Rural Transit Assistance Program,
  www.nationalrtap.org

Of course, to get to the public transportation, we **walk**!

INCREASING DAILY STEPS

Remember that we need about 10,000 steps a day for an active lifestyle. Here are some more ways to increase daily steps:

Daily Habits

- Park in the far back of the parking lot so the walk to the door is longer.
- Get off the bus a stop or two before your usual stop, and walk the rest of the way.
- Use the workplace entrance that is the farthest from your parking spot or bus stop, and walk through the building to your work area.
- Don't just stand—pace; when waiting for the bus, waiting at an elevator, or in other waiting situations, pace around rather than just standing.
- Circle the room when waiting for meetings to start.
- When at work, use the farthest reasonable option for restroom, copy machine, water fountain, and break room.
- Take the stairs rather than the elevator, especially for one to three floors—both up and down.
- When making a phone call, stand up and pace around while talking.
- Rather than using phone or email, walk to a co-worker's office or neighbor's house and converse face-to-face.
- When people stop to talk with you, make it a moving meeting and walk around together while chatting.
- Hide the TV remote and walk to the TV to change channels.
- During TV commercials, get up and walk around the house.

- When doing errands, park in a central location, and walk to all your destinations.

- Return the shopping cart all the way into the store after grocery shopping.

- Use drive-throughs less often; instead, park and walk into the bank or fast-food place.

Short Dedicated Walks

- March in place for several minutes; every 30 minutes, get up from your desk or easy chair and walk in place for 1 to 5 minutes, stretching your arms, shoulders, and neck.

- Before and/or after eating lunch, take a 10-minute walking break.

- Walk the dog.

- Review your usual trips in the car. Could you walk instead of drive to any of your usual destinations, such as the post office?

- When transporting your children to and from sports or other activities, dedicate 10 to 20 minutes to walk around after dropping them off or before picking them up.

- When waiting at the airport, secure your bags and take a good walk around the terminal area.

In other words, make an effort to **just get moving**—up off the couch and into a more active lifestyle. Your body will reward you by running on all cylinders.

PRACTICING WHAT I PREACH

"Pat," you may ask, "what do you do for physical activity?" Since returning from Venezuela, where I walked most places or, at least, to and from buses, taxis, or the subway, I eventually purchased a NordicTrack Cross Country Skier that I have used for about 12 years. It gives me an indoor choice for exercise if it is too hot, cold, or rainy outside. It also combines aerobic and resistance training. There are many similar products on the market ranging from steppers to treadmills to ellipticals and more. I like to walk or work out on the skier most days for about one hour (I estimate that to be 6,000 steps) and alternate with strength training—either free weights or a home weight machine. I exercise using a 20-minute vigorous aerobic workout video on the days I don't have an hour for physical activity. I noticed that when I crossed the 50-year milestone, I had to add strength training to aerobic exercise just to keep my weight normal. I am not fanatical, but I try to do some intentional exercise every day. I average five to six days a week. But life happens, so when I have to go a few days without my usual intentional exercise because of a demanding schedule, I go up and down the stairs at school several times a day or walk around campus to get in extra steps and sunshine! Since I know approximately how many steps I take in 5 minutes (I estimate 500), I know how long I need to walk to get to 10,000 steps a day. When time allows, my husband and I walk or hike together.

Everyone is different. There are so many activities that can keep us active. My husband likes to jog outside and lift weights. Some people prefer active games or team sports. To each his own—just make sure significant movement happens every day!

In the biochemistry of our bodies, the presence of oxygen is necessary to burn calories. Increased physical activity and exercise not only decrease incidence of stress-related diseases like heart disease, cancer, and diabetes, but also improve overall physical and emotional health. Increased lean body mass (muscle mass) and improved lung capacity make our bodies more efficient at burning the calories we eat and the calories that are stored in our bodies as carbohydrate and fat! This, in turn, raises our basal metabolic rate. So if we build lean body mass and increase lung capacity and practice deep breathing to bring in more oxygen—then even at rest, we expend more calories. What a deal!

REMEMBER!

For physical activity/exercise, choose the following:

- Common chores
- Sports activities
- Aerobic activity (intentional)
- Flexibility exercises
- Strength or resistance exercises
- Added daily activity for 10,000 steps

Remember: Most importantly, just get moving!

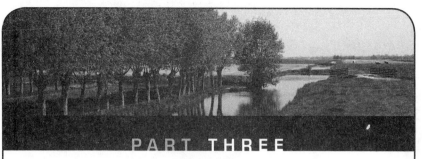

PART THREE
REST

*"Come to me, all you who are weary and burdened,
and I will give you rest. Take my yoke upon you and
learn from me, for I am gentle and humble in heart,
and you will find rest for your souls."*
—Matthew 11:28–29

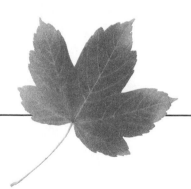

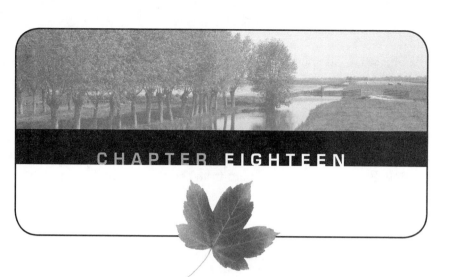

CHAPTER EIGHTEEN

IN EVERYTHING
BY PRAYER

*After [Jesus] had dismissed [the crowd], he went up
on a mountainside by himself to pray.*
—Matthew 14:23

WE have seen how healthy foods and activity can reduce risk of disease and stress in our bodies. In the next few chapters, we will explore how rest (prayer, meditation, and relaxation) can do the same, so that these marvelous bodies God made can function as they were intended to for His glory. We will see how negative thoughts, emotions, and fears, which are all sources of stress, can be reduced through rest—prayer, meditation, and relaxation.

This was God's plan from the beginning. During the Creation, God set aside one day out of seven for rest; He Himself rested when He was finished. He walked in the garden with Adam and Eve. When God gave Moses the Ten Commandments, He repeated His intention for us to remember the Sabbath day—a day of no work, a day of rest. Needing rest does not make us weak or unproductive. Rest is part of God's plan from the time of the Creation.

PRAYER, AN ASPECT OF REST

One of the most significant aspects of rest is **prayer.** A body of scientific research is beginning to show what believers have known for centuries—that the mind and spirit (prayer and meditation) affect the physical body! Participating in the act of prayer, or knowing that others are praying for us, can make a positive difference in our health. Of course, we don't pray as some self-serving effort to benefit ourselves—we pray because of our love for God. Because God is gracious and because God is our true home, prayer returns us to a sense of rest and peace and brings about many other positive effects.

Prayer is the exchange of our sin and daily stress for God's forgiveness, grace, hope, faith, and love. To pray is to rest, simply because we have to focus on God alone. Sometimes prayer may feel like the hardest thing to do, but that doesn't change the fact that prayer puts us in a position of rest in the presence of God.

Prayer is not just asking for the desires of our heart but asking how we fit into God's will, His purpose for our lives. We are His unique creation and fulfill a unique purpose in His eternal plan. Prayer helps us to see ourselves as and where God sees us.

Prayer is considered a *relaxation technique* because it causes a reduction in stress and stress-induced hormones, which helps decrease blood pressure, respiratory rate, pulse rate, and oxygen consumption. In many cases, it creates increased positive feelings and emotions. Negative thoughts, emotions, and behaviors like anger, an unforgiving spirit, and guilt must be confessed through prayer. Many people find that in prayer, God grants them relief and the power to repent and change.

A TIME AND PLACE FOR PRAYER

If we are truly to *"pray without ceasing,"* as Paul exhorts us to do (1 Thessalonians 5:17 KJV), then we should always be in a state of prayer—constantly recognizing God's presence with us. I think Jesus prayed constantly, simply because He and the Father are one (John 10:30; 17:21). There are many examples of Jesus going to a quiet place to pray by Himself, and He instructed His disciples to do the same, as is recorded in Matthew 6:6.

Many people choose to practice prayer through a daily "quiet time," and most of them prefer to have their quiet time in the morning or right before going to bed. A. W. Tozer stressed the importance of meeting with God daily through prayer and meditation. Tozer's book *The Pursuit of God* has meant more to me in my spiritual journey than any other book—outside the Bible, of course! I keep a dog-eared copy with my Bible by my bed. Tozer reminds us that it is only in the very presence of God that we find the rest for our souls that we are all seeking.

God tells us to *"Be still, and know that I am God"* (Psalm 46:10). Praying people usually agree that the best way to commune with God is in a quiet place, alone, with no distractions. Some people have a chosen place for their quiet time that is so well used that simply being there puts them into a state of prayer. But this does not mean that being alone with God is only possible in our usual place or behind closed doors. A person who needs prayer can look for any secluded, quiet place to listen for the still, small voice of God. Many times we find it in places we do not expect.

The prophet Elijah, running for his life, went into a cave to spend the night. In the silence of that cave, God spoke to him. He was told to go out and wait for the presence of the Lord to pass by. He waited. God was not in the terrible wind that arrived and tore the mountains. He was not in the earthquake or fire that came. God came in a gentle whisper (1 Kings 19:9–13). How can we hear God in our prayertime if we are not still and quiet? We must be focused on connecting with the will of God and listening for the voice of God.

JOURNALING DURING PRAYERTIME

Journaling personal prayers and thoughts during prayer and meditation is a proven stress reducer. Expressing thoughts and feelings in writing is recognized as an effective stress management technique in the secular world—doing it while conversing with our Heavenly Father makes it even better!

To begin doing this, place a notebook and pen near your favorite place to pray. Begin recording prayers (things you say to God). It doesn't have to be word for word. Record things God says to you. These may come as streaming or recurring thoughts, or they may come through Scripture. Record requests you make and, later, how those requests are answered. Write down songs to God. Record what the Holy Spirit teaches you through the Scriptures. Record how God is working in your life and the lives of your family members. A prayer journal helps you remember God's words to you, given directly through prayer and through the Bible as you meditate on it.

Examples of writing out prayers and answers to prayers are abundant in Scripture—in the Psalms, Habakkuk, other books of the prophets, and the Book of Revelation. This kind of journaling brought about many of the books included in the Bible.

After the New Testament times, early church fathers continued the practice of writing during prayer and meditation on the Bible. Ancient patterns of sacred reading and contemplative praying are ways to pray through Scripture. We will discuss these methods in more detail in the next chapter on meditation.

PRAYING THE PSALMS

In the Book of Psalms, David gave us wonderful examples of writing out the cry of one's heart to God. He wrote down his prayers and songs to God. He was honest and spared no emotion. These psalms became both a written prayer book and a songbook for the Jewish people. Through the centuries, observant Jews have used Scriptures, especially these psalms, in prayer as they pray at least three times a day. Acts 4:23–30 gives an example of praying a psalm in the early church in the Jewish tradition. Psalms have continued to be a part of the prayers of the church, especially in monastic life and church liturgy. Praying God's Word, the Bible, in a strict sense includes quoting it and using it in our prayers. God responds to His own Word. It will not return to Him empty, but will accomplish what He desires and achieve the purpose for which He sent it (Isaiah 55:11).

One of the best books on praying the psalms is by theologian Dietrich Bonhoeffer. It's called *Psalms: The Prayer Book of the Bible*. Bonhoeffer, you may remember, was a pastor in Germany during World War II and was put to death by the Nazis for participating in a plot on Hitler's life. His book on Psalms guides the Christian to the Scriptures for lessons in how to pray. The book also gives some general background on the history and use of the Book of Psalms as the prayer book of the Bible. In the main part of the book, he presents one possible system of categorizing the psalms according to their petitions, and also points out that they can be organized according to the petitions of the Lord's Prayer. He also shows us how the psalms are to be prayed **in Christ**, of whom they also testify (Luke 24:44).

The psalms reflect every human emotion, but they are emotions seen in relationship to God. Every psalm was written in the presence of God. The psalms teach us how to be honest before God. Being honest before God when praying, especially about negative thoughts, attitudes, emotions, and actions, blesses beyond measure: *"Do not be anxious about anything, but in everything, by prayer and petition, with thanksgiving, present your requests to God. And the peace of God, which transcends all understanding will guard your hearts and your minds in Christ Jesus"* (Philippians 4:6–7).

PATTERNS OF PRAYER

Resources on prayer and how to pray are almost unlimited. One well-known and loved prayer model is the ACTS pattern. To pray using this pattern, simply remember these words that form the acrostic **ACTS**:

A Adoration
C Confession
T Thanksgiving
S Supplication

Begin praying by expressing your adoration to God; next, confess your sins; then thank Him for what He has done and present your supplications, or requests, to Him. David, a man after God's own heart, gave us two beautiful examples of prayers that include adoration, confession, thanksgiving, and supplication in Psalms 32 and 51.

Another often-practiced prayer pattern is to use each section of the Lord's Prayer as a prompt for praise, hope, dependence, forgiveness, and goodness. Since this was the prayer Jesus used to teach the disciples how to pray, it must be a good one for us! Using the King James Version, it works like this:

> *Our Father which art in heaven,*
> *Hallowed be thy name* (praise).
> *Thy kingdom come.*
> *Thy will be done in earth, as it is in heaven* (hope).
> *Give us this day our daily bread* (dependence).
> *And forgive us our debts,*
> *as we forgive our debtors* (forgiveness).
> *And lead us not into temptation,*
> *but deliver us from evil* (goodness).
> —Matthew 6:9–13 (KJV, with prayer pattern
> response added in parentheses)

Both of these patterns are simple enough for even children. Many others are available—just do a Web search for the phrase *prayer pattern*.

BLESSINGS OF PRAYER

Prayer, whether intentional or unceasing, is our connection to God through the Holy Spirit. It is our way of hearing and seeing what God wants us to know and do. As we listen to the Holy Spirit, who intercedes for us in prayer, we find God's will for our lives. Romans 8:26–27 reminds us that many times, we don't even know what to pray for; but the Holy Spirit does. He searches our hearts and knows our mind and speaks for us in accordance with God's will. How amazing is that?

> Blessed is the soul who hears the Lord speaking within her, who receives the word of consolation from His lips. Blessed are the ears that catch the accents of divine whispering, and pay no heed to the murmurings of this world. Blessed indeed are the ears that listen, not to the voice which sounds without, but to the truth which teaches within. Blessed are the eyes which are closed to exterior things and are fixed upon those which are interior. Blessed are they who penetrate inwardly, who try daily to prepare themselves more and more to understand mysteries. Blessed are they who long to give their time to God, and who cut themselves off from the hindrances of the world.
>
> Consider these things, my soul, and close the door of your senses, so that you can hear what the Lord your God speaks within you.
> —Thomas à Kempis, *The Imitation of Christ*

REMEMBER!

Prayer brings power!

- When praying, find a quiet place to be alone.
- Be still.
- Be honest with God.
- Listen intently for His voice.
- Try keeping a prayer journal.
- Set a regular time and place for prayer.
- Try praying the psalms.

Remember: God is waiting to hear from you.

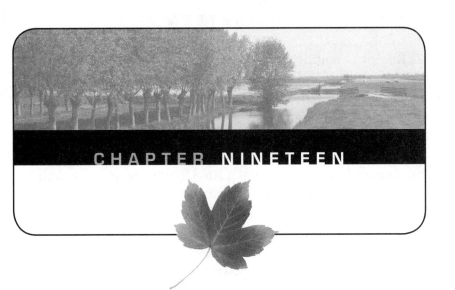

CHAPTER NINETEEN

MEDITATE ON GOD'S PRECEPTS

———————•———————

May the words of my mouth and the meditation of my heart
be pleasing in your sight,
Oh LORD, my Rock and my Redeemer.
—Psalm 19:14

Open my eyes that I may see wonderful things in your law.
Your hands made me and formed me;
give me understanding to learn your commands.
—Psalm 119:18, 73

MANY Christians are devoted to the practice of prayer, but do not consider themselves to be involved in meditation at all. But actually, it is hard to separate prayer and meditation. It has been said that if prayer is talking to God, then meditation is listening to Him.

Recent scientific studies that have verified the health benefits of prayer and meditation come from a variety of notable sources, including the National Institutes of Health, Centers for Disease Control and Prevention (CDC), Harvard Medical School, Cooper Institute for Aerobics Research, Johns Hopkins University, and Duke University. Well-regarded centers and institutes dedicated to research related to spirituality and health are sponsored by some of these institutions, among many others. Prayer and meditation have been shown to offer specific health benefits, mainly involving the reduction of stress response in our bodies. In addition to calming us down and making us feel good, meditation has been shown to sharpen mental activity and change brain structure.

Although science is exploring the benefits of prayer and meditation, many medical doctors still find the mind/body connection and alternative (or complementary) medicine to be a foreign concept. But through personal experience alone, we recognize that our bodies respond to the way we think, feel, and act. When we are stressed, anxious, or upset, our bodies try to tell us that something isn't right. For example, high blood pressure or a stomach ulcer might develop after a particularly stressful event, such as the death of a loved one.

The following may be physical signs that emotional health is out of balance: back pain, chest pain, or general aches and pains; headaches or extreme tiredness; constipation, diarrhea, or upset stomach; change in appetite and unusual weight gain or loss; trouble sleeping; sweating, light-headedness, or heart palpitations; and sexual problems. Poor emotional health can weaken the immune system, making the development of colds and other infections more likely during emotionally difficult times. Also, when feeling stressed, anxious, or upset, we may not take care of our health as well as we should. We may not feel like exercising, eating healthy foods, or even taking medicine that the doctor prescribes.

You may not be used to talking to your doctor about such feelings or problems in your personal life that are causing emotional distress, but it is important to be honest with your doctor if you are having these feelings or experiencing excessive stress.

CALMING EFFECT OF DEEP BREATHING

Stress reduction related to meditation starts with calming the body and mind. One way to calm the body and mind is to sit quietly and still, and concentrate on breathing slowly and deeply—in other words, **practice deep breathing.**

Chronic stress can lead to a restriction of the connective and muscular tissue in the chest. Due to rapid, shallow breathing, the chest does not expand as much as it would with slower, deeper breaths, and much of the air exchange occurs at the top of the lung tissue towards the head. This results in **chest breathing.** To determine if you are a chest breather, place one hand on your chest and the other hand on your abdomen. As you breathe, see which hand rises first—that tells you whether you are a chest or abdominal breather.

Abdominal breathing is also known as **diaphragmatic breathing.** The diaphragm is a large muscle located between the chest and the abdomen. When it contracts, it is forced downward, causing the abdomen to expand.

Deep breathing leads to improved stamina, both in the body's resistance to disease and in athletic activity. Remember that one of the benefits of aerobic activity is increased lung capacity, which increases oxygen consumption in the body through the blood as we inhale and increases release of carbon dioxide through the lungs as we exhale.

Like blood flow, the flow of lymph, which is rich in immune cells, is improved with deep breathing. By expanding the lungs' air pockets and improving the flow of blood and lymph, abdominal breathing also helps prevent infection of the lungs and other tissues. Blood flow carries nutrients and ample amounts of oxygen into the capillaries throughout the body, whereas a healthy lymphatic system carries destructive toxins away from the body tissues. Proper breathing enhances these exchanges.

Deep breathing can eventually deliver many of the benefits of aerobic exercise, including weight loss. Though not a substitute for exercise, deep breathing enhances the benefits of any form of physical activity. Deep breathing alone increases the resting metabolic rate by increasing oxygen capacity. Increased oxygen in the cells helps the body burn extra fat. Deep breathing provides more oxygen to the digestive system also, improving the absorption of nutrients in the body.

Deep breathing is an excellent tool to stimulate the *relaxation response*, the meditation-elicited physiological response that Harvard cardiologist Herbert Benson was the first to note. All forms of meditation, in which the mind becomes quiet and focused, initiate this innate physiological response that is the opposite of the body's stress or fight-or-flight response. Abdominal breathing is an important part of the relaxation response, which results in less tension and an overall sense of well-being.

To begin deep breathing, first, slow down your breathing. Next, force out as much breath as possible from the lungs. Then, breathe in deeply through the nose, expand the abdomen, hold that breath as long as possible, and finally, slowly, slowly exhale through the nose until it seems no breath is left. It is important to get out all that carbon dioxide.

Nose breathing is important when deep breathing. When we inhale through our nose, the hairs that line our nostrils filter out particles of dust and dirt that can harm our lungs. The mucous membranes prepare the air for our lungs by warming and humidifying it. Over time, this filtering and humidification process helps protect our lungs from the damage. Some researchers believe that excessive mouth breathing can cause associated hyperventilation and can result in asthma, high blood pressure, heart disease, and many other medical problems.

Deep breathing slows down the heart rate. In meditative or contemplative prayer, focusing the thoughts while deep breathing can add meaning to this exercise. Focus on "breathing in" thoughts of God with the oxygen in the air, and then "breathe out" anxieties and problems with the carbon dioxide. Prayer is spiritual breathing. Prayers or Scripture or hymns can be recited silently while breathing. This is the basic prayer-breathing relaxation exercise.

Deep breathing and prayer, of course, can be done anywhere, not just during a quiet time. I deep breathe during church—but no one can see me doing it because of my choir robe! Deep breathing can be practiced any time we are still, like while stopping at a red light, watching TV, commuting on the train or subway, or working at the computer. Just think *deep breathe!*

DISCERNMENT IN CHOICE OF MEDITATION TECHNIQUE

Scientific studies have measured many physical and psychological benefits of meditation that leads to relaxation through reduced stress. Meditative techniques separated from Christian spirituality also reduce stress when used for physical relief alone. In general, for the Christian, meditation and relaxation practices that come from Hinduism or Buddhism and other Eastern or New Age religions would be not only inappropriate, but also dangerous. Meditative practices like yoga, T'ai Chi, and Pilates are very effective relaxation techniques. However, practicing these exercises must be for the physical postures alone and not for any religious or philosophical teachings.

Christians must use spiritual discernment in this area (Hebrews 5:14; Colossians 2:8). There are Christian alternatives and variations to many of these exercises that are very beneficial in promoting both physical and psychological health related to stress reduction. A Christian alternative to yoga is promoted by Laurette Willis, founder of PraiseMoves (*www.praisemoves.com*). There are many Christian associations for T'ai Chi as well as for other Chinese martial arts like karate and Tae Kwon Do. Books related to Christian meditation, relaxation techniques, and martial arts are available in abundance. It is interesting that research shows that spiritual meditation is actually more effective in reducing stress that secular meditation.

All of these stress-reducing techniques have been researched by various institutes, and ongoing research may be found at their Web sites. Check these out:

- Mind/Body Medical Institute, *www.mbmi.org*
- National Center for Complementary and Alternative Medicine, National Institutes of Health, *http://nccam.nih.gov*
- Center for Spirituality, Theology and Health at Duke University, *www.dukespiritualityandhealth.org*

PRAYER AND MEDITATION TOGETHER

Jesus made intentional prayertimes a priority in His life. If He did, then how much more should we! In a daily practice of an intentional prayertime, the ideal situation is to be alone, be quiet, and be still. This, in itself, implies meditation—in this stillness, we focus our mind on God. Many people also spend their prayertime with an open Bible.

Although Bible study should be a part of quiet time, **meditation on the Scriptures** is different from an intellectual endeavor. Intellectual study also has its place in our Christian life. But in reading and meditating on the inspired Word of God, we are listening for God to speak to us. Meditation focuses on Jesus through prayer or specific Bible verses. Either way, we are listening for Him. Revelation 3:20 says that Jesus Christ stands at the door (of our hearts) and knocks. If anyone hears His voice and opens the door, He will come in. Again—as with prayer—in meditation, we must be still, we must be quiet, we must be listening.

When we meditate on God's Word, the Holy Spirit draws us into a deeper knowledge and understanding and love of God. This is where prayer and meditation overlap. Meditation over a certain passage may become a prayer. To meditate in Scripture, we must read slowly. We may even choose to memorize it. This allows us to better internalize and personalize the passage.

When we read the Scriptures slowly and prayerfully, allowing them to sink into our hearts, we listen to the Word of God speaking to us **now**. The early Christians used to pray in a method of prayer called **sacred reading**. It was called sacred reading not just because they believed the words of Scripture were inspired, but because they believed that as they read the words, they too would be inspired by the God who inspired the words in the first place. Sacred reading was introduced to the West by the Eastern Christian mystic John Cassian early in the fifth century. The sixth-century *Rule of St. Benedict*, which guided Benedictine and Cistercian monastic practice, continued the practice of sacred reading. These monastic orders and others still prescribe daily periods for sacred reading. In recent decades, however, this ancient tradition has been revitalized by both Catholics and Protestants. Sacred reading involves a progression through reading, meditation, prayer, and contemplation.

In addition to sacred reading, **contemplative prayer** has also been practiced through the centuries from the times of the early church, mainly through the monastic orders. In Christian circles, the terms *meditation* and *contemplation* may be used interchangeably. This practice is characterized by inner and outer silence and solitude. It is waiting in silence for God to speak to us. Contemplative prayer or meditation can be enriched by a tangible aid like a journal, beads, a labyrinth (a pathway for prayerwalking)—always with the purpose of focusing and concentrating attention on praying. These tools lend order to a quiet time to keep us away from distractions in our own minds. They have no other meaning or special significance. Some have even laid out a labyrinth or rocks in their garden like prayer beads to help them pray as they walk among flowers and vegetables. What better way is there to meditate on God's goodness to us?

During contemplative prayer, as in times of sacred reading or any quiet time, we must be sure that **it is God** who is communicating with us. That may sound way out there, but remember that we are in a spiritual battle struggling against the forces of good and evil. John reminds us in 1 John 4:1–4 that we must test the spirits to see whether they are from God. Any insight or instruction that comes during a time of meditation must be in line with what the revealed Word of God teaches; it must pass the test of Christian community; and it must reflect what we know about God through the person of His Son, Jesus. Often meditation serves to bring to mind the very things that we have learned through these other sources of revelation. If an insight does not pass these tests, doubt it! God doesn't lead us in ways that are inconsistent with His Word.

The New Testament offers many examples of **repetitive prayers** used in meditation or contemplation. These were not the *"vain repetitions"* of the pagans (Matthew 6:7), but genuine cries of the heart to God. Luke 18:13 describes a tax collector who, in humble remorse, prayed, *"God be merciful to me a sinner."* This prayer actually became part of the repetitive prayer of the early church called the Jesus Prayer. This repetitive prayer, "Lord Jesus Christ, Son of the living God, have mercy on me, a sinner," like the Jewish Shema, is designed to be said over and over again, until it becomes part of the act of breathing, internalizing a sense of the love of Jesus deep within. Used especially in the Orthodox church, but others as well, this is just one prayer that can be used in Christian meditation or contemplation.

Early monks began to count repetitive prayers by placing stones in their pockets or knots on a rope. This tradition evolved into prayer beads. Prayer beads have not been traditionally used by the Protestant church; however, the recent interest in contemplative prayer and meditation has introduced the tradition of prayer beads into evangelical circles. In the 1980s, Anglicans rediscovered the benefits of prayer beads as an aid in contemplative prayer to engage not only the mind but also the body in prayer and meditation.

Sacred reading, contemplative prayer, and other methods of Christian meditation have been criticized in some evangelical circles for being too close to New Age; however, just because we call focusing on God *meditation* does not mean that it has anything to do with New Age meditation. Meditation was a trusted part of Christian practice long before New Age philosophy came around. Just because it's possible to do a good thing the wrong way doesn't mean we should never do it the right way again! Besides, the Bible urges us to meditate on God's Word (Joshua 1:8, for instance).

There are specific benefits to meditating on Scripture and repeating it over and over, resulting in memorization. Repeating God's Word ingrains it in us until it becomes a part of us. The regular Jewish daily prayer was the Shema, which starts like this: *"Hear, O Israel: The LORD our God, the LORD is One. Love the LORD your God with all your heart and with all your soul and with all your strength"* (Deuteronomy 6:4–5). By Jesus's day, it had already sunk deep into the lives of the Jewish people as not only a formula to be repeated three times a day but a statement of faith—as habitual and as vital as breathing.

Christian meditation is an active thought process given to the study of the Word—praying over it, asking God to give understanding by the Spirit, putting it into practice in daily life, and allowing it (the Word, Scriptures) to become what we do as we go about our daily activities. This causes spiritual growth and maturing in the things of God as taught by His Holy Spirit indwelling each of us as believers. We come into the rest of God as we meditate on Him alone. There must be less of us and more of Him.

> Grant me, most sweet and loving Jesus, to rest in You above every other creature, above all health and beauty, above all glory and honor, above all power and dignity, above all knowledge and precise thought, above all wealth and talent, above all joy and exultation, above all fame and praise, above all sweetness and consolation, above all hope and promise, above all merit and desire, above all gifts and favors You give and shower upon me, above all happiness and joy that the mind can understand and feel, and finally, above all angels and archangels, above all the hosts of heaven, above all things visible and invisible, and above all that is not You, my God.
> —Thomas à Kempis, *The Imitation of Christ*

REMEMBER!

Practice moments of meditation:

- Meditation and prayer may be practiced together during a Christian's daily quiet time.

- Meditation techniques like deep breathing may be practiced for physical and psychological health.

- Deep breathing can increase lung and oxygen capacity to eventually increase resting metabolic rate.

- Meditation in the presence of God helps make us more like Him.

- Repeating God's Word ingrains it in us until it becomes a part of us.

- We come into **the rest of God** as we meditate on Him alone.

Remember: Meditation is healing—physically, emotionally, and spiritually.

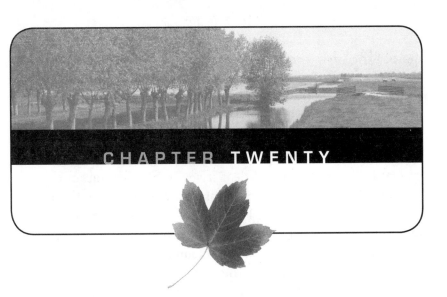

CHAPTER TWENTY

MY FATHER'S WORLD

—————————●—————————

O LORD, our Lord,
how majestic is your name in all the earth!...
When I consider your heavens, the work of your fingers,
the moon and the stars,
which you have set in place,
what is man that you are mindful of him,
the son of man that you care for him?
—Psalm 8:1, 3–4

ONE of my favorite things about living in South America was how much time we spent outdoors. Venezuela is literally one of the most beautiful countries anywhere just because of the different climates. It has everything: thousands of miles of tropical coastline, rain forests, Andean mountains, plains, jungle, and even desert! Because the temperature averages about 75 degrees most of the year, it really is like perpetual spring there. Flowers are everywhere. Poinsettias grow like trees. Bougainvillea can be seen covering the walls of houses. Hibiscus, bromeliads—the list goes on. But the best are the wild orchids in season.

Windows are always open, so birds, birds, and more birds are heard! It's easy to forget how beautiful and enjoyable it is until you go back and see it and hear it again. Standing at an open window or being outside to see and hear the parrots fly over makes me cry every time. I love it, and I miss it. My time spent in Venezuela is probably why I love to be outside now. However, I do hate humidity, so that limits my summertime outside fun in the southeastern US; but in the spring and fall, there is nothing better than to just be outside. I love to eat at a restaurant under an umbrella on the patio or balcony. Sometimes I take my snack or lunch outside and sit on the back steps of the university building where I teach.

The twentieth- and twenty-first-century practice of spending most of the day indoors would seem odd to our ancestors. Recent scientific studies show that being in nature or just looking at pictures of nature can reduce stress and the physical results of stress. A study by Roger Ulrich in 1984 found strong evidence that nature helps heal. Ulrich, a pioneer in the field of therapeutic environments, found that patients recovering from gallbladder surgery who had a window view of trees had significantly shorter hospital stays, voiced fewer complaints, and took less pain medication than those whose window view was a brick wall. This research builds on the work of Harvard naturalist and Pulitzer Prize winner Edward O. Wilson, who coined the term *biophilia* (love of living things). He believes that we have an affinity for nature because we are part of nature.

RESTORED BY NATURE

As part of the natural world, we are connected to and restored by it. The restorative benefits of nature, some experts now believe, can lower blood pressure, boost immune function, and reduce stress. Richard Louv, author of *Last Child in the Woods*, describes the human costs of alienation from nature: diminished use of the senses, attention difficulties, and higher rates of physical and emotional illnesses. He termed the combination of these symptoms *nature deficit disorder*; this condition can be detected in individuals, families, and communities.

Nature deficit can even change human behavior in cities, which could ultimately affect their design, since long-standing studies show a relationship between the absence or inaccessibility of parks and open space with an increase in crime rates, depression, and other urban problems. Scientific studies show that being in a natural environment lowers blood pressure and reduces muscle tension. In fact, just looking at pictures or videos of nature can reduce stress and lessen negative emotions.

We all have our own special way to "get back to nature." One easy way is to open the windows and listen for those birds! Bringing live plants into the house, apartment, or workplace is a great beginning. Believe me—it takes a lot to kill a schefflera plant. Take a lunch outside or sit near the bird feeder for breakfast. Go on a picnic this weekend. Of course, we have already talked about walking or other outdoor activities and sports, which just increase the benefits and joy of being outside.

Another reason to get outside is not only for the sights, smells, and sounds, but for the sunlight itself. Remember that vitamin D is naturally formed in our bodies from sunlight on our skin. Also, research has proven that lack of sunlight actually affects our emotions. For some people, symptoms of depression, sleep disorder, change in behavior, and physical symptoms are so great that they are diagnosed with seasonal affective disorder (SAD). The effects of the seasons on humans were well known in ancient times but were all but abandoned by modern medical practitioners until the 1980s when SAD was first diagnosed. Since a lack of light is the primary problem, it isn't surprising that SAD is more prevalent in winter and that Northerners are at greater risk than Southerners. Light therapy has been an effective treatment for SAD, as well as for milder forms of seasonal depression, often referred to as "winter blues." In fact, most patients improve in less than a week. Symptoms of SAD need to be monitored in children, especially in the northern states during the winter months. Exercise, rest, hugs, kisses, laughter, and other necessities for children that reduce stress hormones also *lessen* the symptoms of SAD, but getting parents, grandparents, and children out into the sunshine is the best way to *prevent* it.

THE JOYS OF GARDENING

One of the best ways to enjoy God's world is to plant a garden! After all, it all started with a garden! A garden does not necessarily have to be neat rows of endless plants that have to be tilled, weeded, sprayed, or mowed. Not at all. Imagine this:

> Picture yourself in a forest where almost everything around you is food. Mature and maturing fruit and nut trees form an open canopy. If you look carefully, you can see fruits swelling on many branches—pears, apples, persimmons, pecans, and chestnuts. Shrubs fill the gaps in the canopy. They bear raspberries, blueberries, currants, hazelnuts, and other lesser-known fruits, flowers, and nuts at different times of the year. Assorted native wildflowers, wild edibles, herbs, and perennial vegetables thickly cover the ground. You use many of these plants for food or medicine. Some attract beneficial insects, birds, and butterflies. Others act as soil builders, or simply help keep out weeds. Here and there vines climb on trees, shrubs, or arbors with fruit hanging through the foliage—hardy kiwis, grapes, and passionflower fruits. In sunnier glades large stands of Jerusalem artichokes grow together with groundnut vines. These plants support one another as they store energy in their roots for later harvest and winter storage. Their bright yellow and deep violet flowers enjoy the radiant warmth from the sky.
> —Dave Jacke and Eric Toensmeier, *Edible Forest Gardens*

An edible forest garden or permaculture is a description of what the Creation's garden would have been. The father of permaculture is Bill Mollison, an Australian who in the 1970s coined the word *permaculture* from a combination of *permanent culture* and *permanent agriculture*, emphasizing that people could provide for their needs by creating self-sustaining relationships among humans, plants, and animals that benefit them all. Mollison based permaculture's principles and practices on this ethical foundation: care for the earth, care for people, and share surplus resources (*www.permaculture.org*).

Whether permaculture, organic gardening, an herb garden, or a flower garden, growing plants and trees in our yard, patio, or window box can bring us joy and make us healthier! In addition, growing our own foods is a wonderful way to help our children and grandchildren see the miracle of life. Many children today don't even know where food comes from. The experience of digging in the dirt and planting seeds that actually turn into food is never forgotten.

GARDENING FOR CHILDREN

Alice Waters, the founder of the Chez Panisse, the original California cuisine restaurant in Berkeley, began the organic revolution that started in the 1970s; she insisted on serving in her restaurant only the fresh local ingredients that were in season. By now, this idea has spread to many neighborhoods with arrival of a natural foods supermarket and a rise in number of small local producers of organic produce, meat, poultry, and dairy products. Fortunately, Alice Waters did not stop with encouraging backyard or small producer gardens; she is now promoting "edible education" for schools. Her idea of a school garden started in one Berkeley school and has now been introduced into the whole Berkeley system.

Of course, some schools have had school gardens for many years; but in the last ten years, with the increase in obesity in children, the National Gardening Association has tried to help schools use gardens as teaching tools. The *www.kidsgardening.com*

Web site has a wealth of resources for gardening with children at home or at school. The Edible Schoolyard, begun by Alice Waters, encourages student participation in all aspects of the gardening experience as they prepare beds, plant seeds and seedlings, tend crops, and harvest produce. Through these activities, students begin to understand the cycle of food production. Vegetables, grains, and fruits grown in soil rich with the compost of last year's harvest are elements of seasonal recipes prepared by students in a school kitchen. Students and teachers sit together to eat and talk at tables set with flowers from the garden. Everyone helps clean up. At the end of each kitchen class, vegetable scraps are taken back to the garden for the compost pile.

This edible education exposes children to food production, ecology, and nutrition and fosters an appreciation of meaningful work and of fresh and natural foods. As Alice Waters herself said of the program, "At first, the kids may not quite believe that they are allowed to have so much fun outside in the garden. But before long, they all know what compost is. And all know what's ripe and what's not ripe and when. This is knowledge they have learned without realizing it from experiences like picking the raspberry patch clean every morning. While they are touching and smelling and tasting, so much information floods in—because they are using all of their senses." Here are some ideas for gardening with children:

- **Let the children help choose the plants.** They will probably choose vegetables and fruits they like to eat. Plant flowers they can cut and bring indoors to arrange.
- **Start small.** Just a few favorite vegetables, fruits, and flowers will be plenty for small hands to help tend.
- **Put the garden where they see it**. A sunny spot where the children play or walk by often is a good choice. The more they see their garden, the more they notice changes. Keep the space to no more than about 4-by-4 feet. Even when no yard is available, a garden can be planted in pots

on a patio or inside on a windowsill—maybe even in the children's rooms.

- **Remember that kids love playing with dirt.** Let them help prepare the soil, even if all they can do is stomp on the clumps. Kid-sized tools allow them to feel even more a part of the project.
- **Identify the plants and the garden.** Mark each plant with the tag or seed packet it came with, so that the children can see what the flowers or vegetables will look like. Also make a sign for the whole garden with the children's names, so everyone else can see whose garden it is.
- **Let them water their garden.** In the fun ranking, playing with water is right up there with playing with dirt. Give the children a small watering can to use on their garden. (Hoses are simply too heavy for little hands to control.) Show them how to gently let the water go right to the roots of the plants.
- **Teach them also about mulching and composting.** Let them spread grass clippings and shredded leaves around their plants to conserve water and help feed the plants. Don't forget to point out any interesting insects.
- **Let the children have control of their garden.** If it's messy, it's their mess. Let them enjoy it and take pride in their own creation.

GARDENING FOR SENIORS

Gardening for seniors is a way to keep active. Many of this generation grew up with a home garden, and a return to the soil is a joy. Following a few suggestions can assist the return to the garden for the older generation.

- **Herbs grow anywhere and are great for seasoning.** Kitchen herb gardens are wonderful for seniors. The more they pinch and pick the herbs, such as basil, parsley, and chives, the more the herbs grow.
- **When creating flowerpots, consider height, filler, and spiller.** Plant a variety that will grow at least two times as

tall as the container, fill in with plants that will grow to no more than half of the height of the taller plants, and then plant a variety that will cascade down.

- **When it comes to annuals, pack them in.** When creating flowerpots, pack the annuals in because they will become root bound and grow up and over the pots. They will provide drama and a beautiful arrangement.
- **Look for equipment that makes the job easier.** Many wonderful tools are available that make gardening easier for anyone, including seniors. Bud-Eze tools, which can be found on the Internet, are a good option, as are Bionic gardening gloves (see *www.bionicgloves.com*). In addition, the Arthritis Foundation (*www.arthritis.org*) has a products and services directory for senior gardeners and others with mobility problems.
- **Garden right outside the front or back door.** Container gardening allows seniors access to flowers or vegetables in one pot and also allows the plants to be placed at a height that make gardening easier for them.
- **Garden with others.** Teaming up with others to garden gives seniors needed companionship.
- **If a senior can't garden anymore, enlist the help of others**. Find someone who might enjoy sharing the work and any produce or flowers from the garden. Contact Home Instead Senior Care (*www.homeinstead.com*) to find a caregiver who would enjoy gardening with that person.

JUST BEING OUTSIDE

Gardening, picking strawberries or blueberries or muscadines, camping, hiking, fishing, birding, viewing the stars, swimming, hunting, participating in winter activities, or relaxing in the hammock—just being outside, no matter what we are doing, reminds us of our Creator God. The following Web sites and books give ideas for outdoor activities to do with family:

- *www.americaoutdoors.com*
- *www.americanhiking.org*
- *The Appalachian Trail Backpacker* by Victoria and Frank Logue
- *Recipes for Roughing It Easy* by Dian Thomas

REMEMBER!

God is a part of all His creation.

- Spend time outdoors every day.

- Listen. God still talks to us through His creation.

- Enjoying nature at any age brings us closer to the God who created it.

- We do see and hear and feel God when we look and listen for Him around us.

- Being in a natural environment reduces stress and the physical damage of stress on the body.

- Lack of sunlight affects the body adversely both physically and emotionally.

- Growing a vegetable or flower garden reconnects us with God's world. And it is even more of a blessing when done with family—children, grandchildren, parents, grandparents.

- What better way is there to enjoy the wholeness that God created for us than to eat, move, and rest under the blue sky, bright sun, and brilliant stars of His world?

Remember: God's world was made for us. Get out and enjoy it!

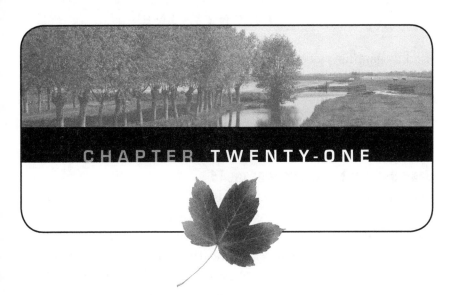

CHAPTER TWENTY-ONE

CHESS, MARBLES, DOMINOES, AND DINNER

●

The apostles gathered around Jesus and reported to him all they had
done and taught. Then, because so many people were coming and
going that they did not even have a chance to eat, he said to them,
"Come with me by yourselves to a quiet place and get some rest."
—Mark 6:30–31

JESUS playing checkers? Well, maybe not, but that's
not beyond the realm of possibility. In Bible times, as
today, people of the Middle East spent a lot of time
playing checkers, backgammon, chess, and similar
games. In almost every excavation of ancient sites
in the Middle East, gaming boards have been found.
Boards were often of limestone, divided into squares,
and pebbles, small stones, bones, or pieces of clay were

used as gaming pieces. My guess is that even if Jesus and His disciples never touched a marble, their time away together was enjoyed, as they relaxed, told stories, fellowshipped, and dined together. Jesus knew the value of time spent with those He loved.

HANG OUT, BUT NOT IN FRONT OF THE TV

Spending time with spouse, friends, or family in conversation, playing games, or just hanging out is time well spent. This could mean some time in front of the tube watching a movie or sporting event, but most of the time, TV time is **wasted** time. I am not just preaching to the choir here. I could be a serious TV addict myself. Abundant research shows that time in front of the TV equals inactivity, a fact that couch potatoes know and show full well! TV time also correlates with obesity, sleep problems, and behavior problems in children and adolescents, including aggressiveness and violence. Consider these tips provided by the American Academy of Pediatrics that will help you tame that TV monster for your children or grandchildren:

- Limit TV viewing to one to two hours a day. No watching TV while doing homework.

- Don't leave the TV on as background noise. Help your child decide which shows to watch, and turn on the TV for only those shows.

- Watch TV with your child, and talk about what you see. For very young children, explain the difference between commercials and TV shows. Explain that TV characters are not real.

- Be careful about what you watch in the presence of your child; news and other shows often contain violence.

- Talk about the messages TV shows are sending.

- Help your child learn to resist commercials. Explain that commercials are supposed to make people want things.

- Consider limiting your child's viewing to public television programs or children's videos.

- Don't let TV become a habit. Help your child think of other things to do, such as playing, reading, or working on art projects.
- Practice what you preach. Limit your own TV viewing, and choose what you watch carefully.
- Be clear and consistent about the rules.

Too much TV and video-game time can actually affect brain development. Research has shown that cognitive learning is adversely affected with TV viewing, especially in children younger than three years. The American Academy of Pediatrics suggests that TV be limited in young children because of the increased risk of attention deficit disorder (ADD) and attention deficit hyper-activity disorder (ADHD). Provide children books or ideas for fun activities. One good series of books for children is the "I Spy" collection by Jean Marzollo and Walter Wick. Also check out *www.funattic.com*. When TV viewing is limited, it gives children a chance to use their imaginations. What could be better than a large box for a rainy day! For those who grew up with Howdy Doody, Captain Kangaroo, and Mister Rogers, TV addiction may not seem to be a problem, but for our sports, soap opera, and reality TV culture, you can bet that more time could be spent developing our brains no matter what our age is. For more ideas about giving the TV a boot, go to *www.tvturnoff.org* and *www.limitv.org*.

THE AGING BRAIN

Aging research has shown that we have to use our brains to keep them functional. As we age, we all have our "senior moments" when we look for the glasses that are on our heads or forget what we just came into a room for. As we age, forgetfulness happens! Of course, when progressive memory loss and confusion begin to affect everyday life skills, then these symptoms go beyond the norm. Brain atrophy begins in middle age. Just like muscles in our body, as we age, we must use it or lose it. That's why participating in quiet activities that actually build brain cells is a better idea than just being a couch potato, no matter what size the potato!

Not only is our brain what we eat, it is what we think! Staying mentally active while aging not only keeps us from losing brain cells and connections, but it actually helps build new ones! The term *lifelong learning* is not just a phrase to torture recent college graduates, but a reality if we are to stay mentally sharp rather than experience dotage. If enrolling in a computer or Spanish class seems like a little too much, begin with some of these brain-building activities:

- **Lose the calculator.** Next time you balance your checkbook, do it in your head or on paper. Figure the tip in your head at the restaurant.
- **Keep the grocery list hidden.** Visualize the refrigerator and pantry to see what's in stock. Just before checking out, check your list to see if you've remembered everything.
- **Do crossword puzzles and word jumbles daily.**
- **Play Sudoku.** This number puzzle has quite a following and is apparently addictive.
- **Play board games and word games.**
- **Learn a new word or Bible verse each week.** Review these as a family each day.
- **Recite the alphabet backwards until you are proficient.** Try this exercise three times a day until you can do the backwards version as quickly as the regular version. This takes work!
- **Read riddle books and try to solve them.** These riddles also make good party icebreakers.
- **Get organized!** Keep your keys in the same place each day. Clean your desk. Straighten your closet. When your life is organized, you spend less time worrying about where things are and other details that cloud the mind. Just the process of organizing clears your mind.
- **Take up a hobby that forces you to think outside the box.** Some examples include learning a foreign language or sign language. Learn how to read music. Make certain to incorporate the newly acquired information into your lifestyle.

- Listen to a different kind of music than usual.
- If you walk or jog, find a new route.
- Write some poetry.

Think up other creative ways to exercise your brain. The point is to just do it—get mentally active. All the information anyone could ever want about board games, card games, puzzles, brain teasers, and all manner of fun can be found at a bookstore or on the Internet—and a good amount can be found in the daily newspaper.

BRAIN EXERCISES

Traditional brain exercises help us focus on specific types of skills. A program called Neurobics suggests ways to make the brain work differently. Some examples of Neurobic exercises are brushing your teeth with the opposite hand, taking a shower or finding your way around the house with eyes closed, listening to a specific piece of music while burning a scented candle, taking a different way home from work, and rearranging your work desk. Many of our day-to-day tasks are done with our brain on autopilot. Neurobics forces the areas of the brain that aren't normally used much to actually go to work. Researchers say strengthening all the areas helps the brain become more flexible and efficient and may help maintain mental agility in old age. Making multisensory associations and doing something novel that is important to you or engaging are the key conditions for a genuine Neurobic exercise. Check out *www.neurobics.com* or the book, *Keep Your Brain Alive: 83 Neurobic Exercises to Help Prevent Memory Loss and Increase Mental Fitness* by Lawrence Katz and Manning Rubin. Other brain games like Brain Age (*www.brainage.com*) are literally like "brain food" according to some researchers, such as those at the Stress Institute (*www.stressinstitute.com*).

Playing games, working puzzles, learning new things, and doing familiar routines differently are just a few activities that you and your family can do together not only to keep minds active and growing, but to bond more closely.

TOGETHER TIME

There is **no substitute for time together**. Hopefully, there are times each day at bedtime or first thing in the morning when you spend a few minutes with each child or other family member to talk, read, or pray together. In regard to time spent, quality is important, but so is quantity. A weekly family night or a date with one child at a time goes a long way toward letting your children know you love them. Include children in your hobbies, such as bowling, coin collecting, fishing, crafts, woodworking, or cooking. A special outing with your child may be going out to dinner and a movie, going skating, spending an afternoon at the lake or beach, taking a hike, going to a sporting event, or stargazing. Your children probably have some interesting suggestions of their own.

Of course, date night with your spouse is nonnegotiable! Many times I combine a date night with a surprise menu for my husband or family.

MEALTIME MAGIC

My idea of fun lifelong learning is trying new ingredients, new foods, and new recipes! One of the favorite food classes I teach is Food, Culture, and Society. Typically, each student takes a different cuisine from around the world and researches the history, customs, meal patterns, ingredients, and so forth. The greatest part of the research is cooking and eating the food. This is much more fun than chemistry lab! We may eat with our hands while sitting on the floor if that is the custom of the particular country we are learning about that day. (Now, I could try that at home. In fact, that is a great idea for the next time we keep the grand-children!) Cooking new recipes from a variety of cultures with new tastes and smells brings fun and learning into the kitchen. Some great ideas can be found in *Stirring Up a World of Fun* by Nanette Goings.

How often have we heard, "The family that prays together stays together." I would be willing to bet that these are the families that also eat together. Maybe family meals don't have to happen every night, but they *are* important. Research has shown that family meals can lead to better physical and mental health for both the adults and the children. Studies show that when meals are eaten at home as a family, more fruits and vegetables are eaten! Eating meals together as a family most or all days is associated with both eating healthier, in general, and decreased risk for obesity. Of course, this is not surprising. Other benefits of the family meal are that children who frequently eat meals with their family tend to do better in school, and they are less likely to be at risk for substance abuse and depression. Family meals are a time for parents and children to talk and share feelings. Miriam Weinstein, the author of *The Surprising Power of Family Meals: How Eating Together Makes Us Smarter, Stronger, Healthier, and Happier*, says that the combination of eating and talking is powerful. Research shows that even eating one meal a week together can make a difference, but that the more frequent, the better. This meal does not even have to be at home, since the important issue is to eat facing each other and not the TV. One of the joys of being in Latin America, Italy, Spain, or France is to observe large families eating together. Relationships and family seem to be so much more important in some cultures than they seem to be here in America. Of course, Americans lived that way a century ago. Our fast-paced society doesn't leave much time for our families or each other. This is where the concept of slow food comes in again. When we take time to enjoy food and fellowship together, something magical happens.

A great way for a family to have fun, learn, and love each other is to cook and eat together when possible. Meals do not have to be elaborate, but they can be when time allows—on the weekends or during school breaks. Cooking together as a family, setting the table, practicing table manners, and even lighting a few candles as my grandchildren love to do—these activities make special memories that last a lifetime. It doesn't even have to be a meal. When our children were small, we participated in a nightly ritual of a cup of raspberry or other fruit tea (without caffeine) with cookies, fruit and cheese, peanut butter, or whatever we could find. My best memories are during the winter when this little party could be held by the fireplace. We always used cups and saucers (not mugs), real milk or cream, and sugar cubes (the children loved those, for some reason). Occasionally, we still have a tea party when we are all together at home. These are the times we learn to listen and share ideas as a family—we get to *know* each other.

MAKES SCENTS TO ME

Cooking and eating together as a family have some unexpected health benefits. Research shows that kitchen aromas reduce anxiety and stress! Imagine that—the smell of cookies or freshly baked bread being good for you! Studies have shown that aromas can increase the oxygen uptake of the brain by almost 30%. Such an increase in brain oxygen can lead to an increased level of activity in the brain, which can have dramatic effects not only on emotions, learning, and attitude, but also on many physical processes of the body, such as immune function, hormone balance, and energy levels. Wow!

Aromatherapy has been practiced for thousands of years. The Greeks, Romans, and ancient Egyptians all used aromatherapy oils. Hippocrates, the father of modern medicine, used aromatherapy baths and scented massage. He used aromatic fumigations to rid Athens of the plague. When inhaled through the nose, odor stimulates the brain to release chemicals like endorphins and serotonin, which can reduce pain, create a sense of euphoria, and relax and energize both mind and body. Inhaled through the nose, fragrances have a powerful effect on our state of mind and physical well-being. Bring on the cinnamon!

Mary Capone shares some ideas in "Kitchen Therapies":

The next time you slice a lemon, orange, or grapefruit, take a moment to inhale its heady fragrance. Citrus odors are great pick-me-ups. They trigger the brain to produce the neurochemical encephalins which creates euphoria and induces a feeling of well-being. In addition, the scent of orange comforts the lonely; lemon keeps you alert; and grapefruit acts as a mild pain reliever.

Bake an apple pie and fill your house with happiness and serenity. The scent of green apples has been found to have a tranquilizing effect helping to reduce stress and anxiety. For an important dinner guest, bake a batch of cinnamon rolls. The scent of these freshly baked rolls have been found to be an aphrodisiac.

Your spice cabinet has medicinal remedies for what ails you. The next time you need an extra dose of confidence or courage, add cinnamon sticks and cloves to a pot of lightly boiling water and make a potpourri. Cinnamon helps relieve anxiety and cloves make you feel less vulnerable and afraid. The aroma of fresh ginger root stimulates digestion, while grated nutmeg sprinkled in dishes can help treat sore muscles and depression.

Buy a bouquet of aromatic flowers [place them in a vase on your kitchen table] and smell them frequently as you pass. Roses can stimulate happiness, ease depression, and relieve stress. Add jasmine to your bouquet to restore a love of life and geraniums to balance hormones.

Growing a garden of herbs on your kitchen windowsill or outdoors can spice up your life as well as your palate. When gathering fresh herbs for your culinary masterpiece, take a moment to break off the ends of the leaves and inhale.

- *Basil* is a great mental stimulant and uplifts the troubled mind and heart.
- *Chamomile,* used in a bowl of steaming water, is good for sunburns, acne, and inflammations of the skin. Chamomile also acts as a digestive aid in tea and is a great remedy for insomnia.
- *Eucalyptus* has the effect of clearing the mind as well as cooling fevers. When you are suffering from a head cold, create a natural vaporizer by

floating eucalyptus leaves in a steaming bowl of water. Cover your head with a towel creating a tent over the bowl and breathe in.

- *Lavender* has so many uses that it is essential for any garden. When inhaled, lavender eases headaches, relieves stress, induces happiness, fights insomnia and irritability, helps sore joints, soothes burns, and fights persistent infections.
- *Lemongrass* combats exhaustion and increases concentration.
- *Marjoram* calms the nerves.
- *Mint leaves* aid digestion while alleviating cramping.
- *Peppermint* helps fight fatigue, forgetfulness and relieves headaches.
- *Rosemary* supports the nervous system.
- *Spearmint* eases grief.
- *Thyme* stimulates the immune system and is great when fighting colds.

(Available at: *www.gaiam.com/retail/gai_content/learn/gai_learnArticle.asp?article_id=52*. Used with permission.)

Whether you are peeling an orange, grating ginger, cooking with fresh herbs, or picking a rose, take a deep breath and **do yourself a "flavor."**

A great book related to kitchen therapy is *Aromatherapy in the Kitchen: Fragrant Foods for Body, Mind and Spirit* by Melissa Dale, Emmanuelle Lipsky, and Kellie Canning.

TIME WELL SPENT

Time spent with those we love is always time well spent. Not only does it draw us closer together, it heals—mind, body, and spirit. When we really take time to think about what is important or what matters most in life, it all boils down to our relationship with God and others. Everything else is just fluff. Take time today.

REMEMBER!

Fun and games bring people together.

- Table and brain games engage the mind and rest the body.
- Cooking and eating together as a family is food for the body and soul.
- Aromatherapy in the kitchen or elsewhere reduces physical stress.

Remember: Take time to have fun with friends and family.

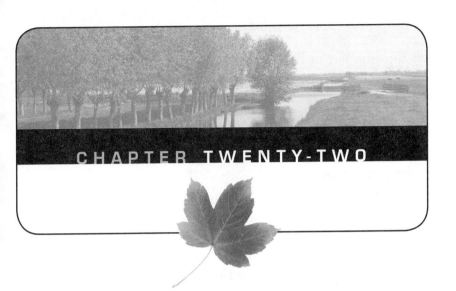

CHAPTER TWENTY-TWO

HUGS, KISSES, AND LAUGHTER

———————●———————

People were bringing little children to Jesus to have him touch them.
—Mark 10:13

A cheerful heart is good medicine.
—Proverbs 17:22

HIPPOCRATES acknowledged touch as one of the oldest healing remedies. Touch is probably older than any other healing tradition. The oldest written records of touch as massage go back 3,000 years to China, but it is much older than that, of course. Touch and the laying on of hands are human tendencies that are inherent. Physicians and healers of all forms and from all cultures have used hands-on manipulation throughout history as an integral part of health-care practice. In the former Soviet countries, Germany, Japan, and China, massage has continued uninterrupted, as massage therapists today work alongside doctors as part of the health-care team. Today, the healing power of touch is an expanding area of research within scientific circles.

IMPORTANCE OF TOUCH

Exercise, meditation, laughter, touch—all these are known to cause the body to release those wonderful endorphins, those stress-relieving hormones.

For many years, research has documented the effect of touch on infants. Infants who have adequate nutrition and no physical problems but do not grow properly are sometimes diagnosed as having nonorganic failure to thrive. Failure to thrive in infants can come from improper feeding or diseases like cystic fibrosis, but research has shown that neglect alone can cause failure to grow and thrive. That is why mother/baby bonding is so important. Recent research has shown that infants and even premature babies who receive infant massage gain more weight, have fewer gastrointestinal problems, and sleep better than infants not massaged.

Physicians are now beginning to diagnose failure to thrive in nursing homes and extended-care facilities. Massage therapy has been shown to reduce the physical and psychological symptoms of stress in those with failure to thrive and to enhance the quality of life for all residents. Touch or massage has been shown to increase blood circulation, improve the lymphatic system, release toxic by-products in the muscles, reduce stress, relieve tension, and increase energy. Touch or massage therapy has also been used successfully in hospice care. In fact, there is a general correlation between the therapy and longer length of life for many patients in hospice care.

So, who have *you* hugged today?

By observation, I have noticed that there are touching families and there are nontouching families. If your family is in the nontouching category, I challenge you to find some family therapy or self-help. *The Five Love Languages* by Gary Chapman is an excellent resource for increasing the number of hugs and kisses in the family.

In *Tools for Raising Responsible Children*, James and Constance Messina describe family affection this way:

> Bonding with children means helping them have a sense of security, being wanted, self-worth, and self-esteem. Bonding is accomplished by hugging children, either physically or verbally. Bonding is the mutual emotional attachment between parents and their children. It is the way in which unconditional acceptance and love are transmitted between them. It creates an emotional connection which provides the sense of security and trust in the family relationship. This sense of being wanted is demonstrated in their mutual ongoing physical and verbal hugging. Bonding is the emotional intimacy with parents which is the basis for their children's future healthy intimate relationships. Appropriate physical touching, holding, caressing, cradling, kissing, massaging, and hugging are all external nonverbal ways of connecting in a bonding way. Verbal recognition, encouragement, reinforcement, statements of gratitude and appreciation, verbal expressions of acceptance, love, and closeness are just a few of the verbal forms of hugging which create a bond with children.
> —James J. Messina, PhD, and Constance M. Messina, PhD, *Tools for Raising Responsible Children* (available at *www.coping.org*)

Amen to that!

In Latin America, the *abrazo* is the hug for everyone—not just your family. If your cultural background is not touchy-feely, don't give up; family affection can be cultivated.

LOVE BUG

And speaking of family affection, the love bug can bring on the endorphins big time! So get huggy and cuddly with your partner to enjoy an endorphin rush. Couples who enjoy an intimate relationship decrease overall stress and improve health, not only physically, but also emotionally. Intimate touch means more than just making love; just making out can turn on the chemical process. When making love, the human body releases endorphins, but also produces chemicals that create stronger feelings of affection between couples; the activity stimulates production of growth hormones that reduce fatty tissue and increase lean muscle; and it burns off more than 100 calories per hour. And remember, absolutely **no** television in the bedroom. Research has shown that couples who **do not** have a TV in their bedroom make love twice as often as those who do! Need I say more?

HAVE A LAUGH

When love is all around, so is laughter. For many years, *Reader's Digest* has insisted that laughter is the best medicine; a book by that title even now declares it. Scientific research is proving just that. Of course, it makes sense: if things that make us happy relieve stress and make us healthier, then laughter certainly should. There are now clubs virtually around the globe that model the laughter clubs of India.

In the United States, the medical world started taking note of the possibilities of therapeutic laughter after Norman Cousins's book *Anatomy of an Illness as Perceived by the Patient* came out in 1979. In it, he describes how watching Marx Brothers movies, *Candid Camera*, and other comedies helped him fight a life-threatening disease of the joints and connective tissue. Now hospitals, nursing homes, and private clubs all around the country are hiring laughter leaders, certified by the Association for Applied and Therapeutic Humor, who teach the healing value of laughter. One of the things Cousins documented was that a ten-minute belly laugh could give him two hours of painless sleep. Many other studies suggest that the ability to manage and conquer pain can largely be predicted by a patient's frame of mind. The physiological effects of a 30-minute to one-hour session of viewing a humorous video have appeared to last up to 12 to 24 hours in some individuals. A friend and colleague at my university was involved in a serious automobile accident two years ago. The type of back injury that he sustained should have killed him. In addition to his tremendous faith and support from his family and friends, he credits humor and a positive attitude for much of his healing.

THE AGING NEED A TOUCH TOO

If any place in the world is in need of hugs, kisses, and laughter, it is the traditional nursing home. One gerontologist, William H. Thomas, hopes to change all that with his Eden Alternative and Green House concepts for extended care.

In the 1990s, Thomas's Eden Alternative concept called for making the sterile atmosphere of the nursing home more like a real home, with plants, pets, and children, and letting residents care more for themselves, with the help of staff.

The Green Houses are family-size homes of ten residents or fewer, each with private bedrooms and baths around a common area, including the kitchen and laundry facility! They have porches and outdoor gardens. All meals are taken together with staff and visitors in a family atmosphere. Quality of life for the elderly has dramatically improved in the Green Houses already in place. Seniors who were in wheelchairs are walking, seniors who were solitary are talking, and seniors who were not eating now have an appetite. The director of the Green House in Tupelo, Mississippi, has reported that through something as simple as enabling Green House residents to smell the bacon cooking, the small pleasures of life are restored. Those small pleasures are what hope and life and love are made of. *"'For I know the plans I have for you,' declares the LORD, 'plans to prosper you and not to harm you, plans to give you hope and a future'"* (Jeremiah 29:11).

REMEMBER!

No man, woman, or child is an island.

- Touch reduces physical stress and is associated with healing.
- Human beings are wired for affection—from birth to death.
- Laughter flows naturally from love and affection.

Remember: Love, affection, touch, and laughter are literally good medicine!

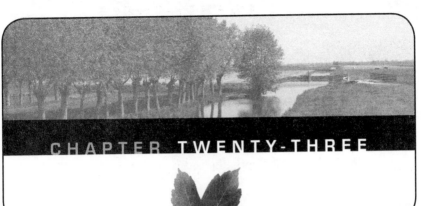

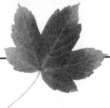

CHAPTER TWENTY-THREE

SWEET DREAMS

———————•———————

I lie down and sleep;
I wake again, because the LORD sustains me.
—Psalm 3:5

I will lie down and sleep in peace,
for you alone, O LORD,
make me dwell in safety.
—Psalm 4:8

SLEEP is as important for good health as proper nutrition and exercise are. Deep sleep and rapid eye movement (REM) sleep (during which dreaming occurs) keep us well by promoting healthy immune function and production of growth hormones and keeping us energized and clear-minded.

Sleep occurs in cycles that last about 90 minutes each. A person may complete five cycles in a typical night's sleep. The amount of sleep necessary to function varies from person to person, with some sleeping only a few hours and others unable to do without a full 10 hours. For good health, most adults need between 7 and 9 hours of sleep a night; children need about 10 to 14 hours of sleep, depending on age.

SLEEP FOR YOUR HEALTH

Sleep affects all aspects of our health. Studies indicate that risk for disease starts to increase when people get less than 6 or 7 hours of sleep a night. Sleep deficit may put the body into a state of high alert, causing the production of stress hormones and inflammation in the body, both of which increase risk factors for obesity, heart disease, stroke, cancer, diabetes, and depression.

One interesting finding suggests that men and women who work night shifts are at higher risk for breast and prostate cancer. Nighttime illumination (bright light) interrupts the body's nocturnal production of the hormone melatonin. Melatonin, which is produced in our body only in the dark, protects our bodies from hormone-related tumors. Decreased production of melatonin increases the risk of those cancers.

Other studies show that lack of sleep increases both plaque in blood vessels and blood pressure. Since blood pressure naturally rises in the morning anyway, insomnia could be a factor in the many heart attacks and strokes that occur early in the morning.

Infectious diseases tend to make us feel sleepy. This probably happens because the chemicals our immune systems produce while fighting an infection are powerful sleep inducers. Sleep may help the body conserve energy and other resources that the immune system needs to fight the infection.

INTERNAL BODY CLOCK

While many aspects of sleep remain a mystery (including exactly *why* we sleep) a body of research is beginning to accumulate to show that not sleeping enough or being awake in the wee hours of the night upsets the body's internal clock, throwing a host of basic bodily functions out of sync.

Our internal body clock is regulated by light and darkness. Our bodies were not made to be working by fluorescent lights or watching the lights of a TV at 3:00 A.M. Before *Midnight Madness* and *Late Show with David Letterman* came along, Ben Franklin probably had the right idea: "Early to bed and early to rise makes a man healthy, wealthy, and wise." Going to bed and getting up at the same time every day—even on weekends—goes a long way toward keeping body rhythms regulated.

The circadian rhythm dips and rises at different times of the day. The strongest sleep drives generally occur between 2:00 and 4:00 A.M. and in the afternoon between 1:00 and 3:00 P.M., although these sleep drive times vary, depending on whether we are a *morning* or *evening* person. The sleepiness experienced during these dips is less intense if we have had sufficient sleep and more intense when we are sleep deprived.

NIX DROWSY DRIVING

Sleepiness while driving—whether due to dip times or sleep deprivation—has been experienced by most all adults. Getting behind the wheel of a vehicle when sleepy is as dangerous as drinking and driving. However, according to a recent poll by the National Sleep Foundation (NSF), 60% of adults licensed to drive say they have driven drowsy in the past year. What that means is that about 118 million people are making our roads more dangerous because they are driving when they are sleepy and less alert than they should be. The National Highway Traffic Safety Administration (NHTSA) conservatively estimates that 100,000 police-reported crashes each year are the direct result of driver fatigue and cause an estimated 1,550 deaths and 71,000 injuries. Virtually everyone is at risk, at times, for drowsy driving. Watch out for these five warning signs:

- Difficulty focusing or keeping eyes open
- Yawning repeatedly
- Trouble remembering the last few miles driven
- Drifting from your lane or hitting a shoulder rumble strip
- Missing traffic signs or exits

If you start to feel tired while driving, find a safe, well-lit area, and stop for a break or for the night. Caffeine can promote short-term alertness, but it takes about 30 minutes for it to enter the bloodstream and provide that effect. Take a 15- to 20-minute nap while waiting for the caffeine to kick in.

SLEEP DEPRIVATION

Let's face it—most Americans just don't get enough sleep in this 24/7 society. Sleep deprivation in America affects people of all ages, from children to older adults. Causes range from **sleep disorders** to simply **poor choices.**

Sleep Disorders

Insomnia or sleep disorders, which may occur intermittently or for several days or months at a time, may be identified with the following:

- Difficulty falling asleep
- Waking frequently during the night
- Waking too early in the morning and not being able to get back to sleep
- Waking feeling unrefreshed
- Falling asleep at inappropriate times
- Abnormal behaviors associated with sleep

Sleep disorders could include sleep apnea, restless leg syndrome, and narcolepsy among others. If you suspect you or a family member has insomnia or a sleep disorder, contact a physician for help. Web sites like *www.sleepfoundation.org* may also be helpful.

Sleep Obstacles

A major obstacle to a good night's sleep in most homes could be the tube in the bedroom. Let's say it again: **No TV in the bedroom!** Lest you think the already stated reasons aren't good enough, here are more! A National Sleep Foundation poll found that 30% of preschoolers and 43% of school-age children have a television in their bedroom. What's more, the National Institute on Media and the Family reported that children with a TV in their bedroom are likely to spend an additional five and a half hours a week watching it. That's about 45 minutes a day that could be better spent reading, playing outside, or sleeping. Most research has centered on the effects of TV on children, but for teenagers and adults, having a TV in the bedroom will likely result in resisting going to bed, having trouble falling asleep, not sleeping as long, and daytime sleepiness. Don't allow a TV in the bedroom! And if you have already allowed it, get it out—out of your room and out of your child's room.

The American Academy of Pediatrics recommends that children's bedrooms be media-free zones. That means no computer, no video games, and, certainly, no TV set. The same rules for adults could improve their sleep experiences.

Our electronic toys—computers and TVs—are not the only obstacles to a good night's sleep. Here are some suggestions for overcoming other obstacles:

- Consume less or no caffeine and avoid alcohol near bedtime.
- Drink less fluid before going to sleep.
- Avoid heavy meals close to bedtime, but don't go to bed hungry either.
- Avoid nicotine.
- Exercise regularly, but do so in the daytime or at least three or more hours before bedtime.
- Don't keep the bedroom too hot.
- Don't bring work-related material or a computer to the bedroom.

- Avoid napping during the day unless limited to 30 minutes or less.
- Avoid the evening news.
- Don't even try to go to sleep if you are completely awake! Duh!
- Don't take your trouble or anger to bed.
- Avoid bright light in the bedroom or bathroom before bedtime.

THE BEDROOM

Now that we've settled some issues about what **should not** be a part of your bedroom, what **should** a room where you spend one-third of your life be like? A bedroom should be a haven, an escape, a private sanctuary; a place for reflection; a place to read, to meditate, to pray, to listen to music, to daydream, to love, to sleep—a sacred retreat. This bedroom invites complete rest of body, mind, and spirit. A bedroom should be a place where all your senses are at home. Soothing colors, soft music, low lighting or candlelight, fragrant flowers, and soft pillows can help reduce the stress of the day. Even if we have no other fresh flowers in the house, I keep roses or other fragrant flowers in our bedroom and bathroom along with candles and favorite CDs. Many times, I use the sitting area in the bedroom for a quiet miniretreat for myself alone or with my husband. I like to read there, nap there, or just listen and watch the birds out of our "wall of windows" in my favorite room of the house. Sometimes I have cheese or peanut butter and crackers and apples or strawberries and milk waiting for Bob when he gets home too late for a real dinner. This is our time to wind down. Time spent this way is better than time spent raising our stress levels listening to the nightly news.

The bedroom is a sanctuary for dreaming and a place where our dreams can begin to come true! Yes, dreaming is good for us. Good dreaming contributes to our psychological well-being by supporting healthy memory and warding off depression. Our brain restructures new memories during sleep, helping us to solve problems and become more insightful.

CHOICES FOR GOOD SLEEPING

Sleep is very simply a basic necessity of life, as fundamental to our physical health and well-being as air, food, and water. If we don't sleep well, or sleep enough, almost every aspect of our lives will suffer. So tonight, **choose** to get a good night's sleep. Here are a few more suggestions for developing a good bedtime routine:

- Establish a regular bedtime and ritual.

- Participate in daily physical activity.

- Keep the bedroom as dark as possible for melatonin production; don't turn on a bright light if you get up at night.

- Keep the bedroom at about 70 degrees year-round.

- Take a soaking hot bath or sauna before bedtime—not a shower!

- At least an hour before bedtime, have a light snack that provides complex carbohydrates and protein containing tryptophan. (Tryptophan is an amino acid that aids in serotonin production; serotonin turns into melatonin when we are asleep in the dark.) Examples of good bedtime snacks are pasta with Parmesan cheese, cheese or peanut butter with crackers, hummus on pita bread, or cereal and milk. Warm milk with cinnamon or nutmeg and a little stevia or honey is great! Calcium in dairy products also aids in melatonin production.

- Drink herbal teas to sooth and relax you—chamomile, lavender, lemon balm, or passionflower and herbal blends.

- Don't forget aromatherapy! Herbal baths, sachets, or essential oils can provide the benefits of lavender, sandalwood, sage, and many other herbs.

- Stop studying an hour or two before trying to go to sleep.

- Keep a pad and pen or tape recorder by the bed, so when thoughts cross your mind that must be remembered in the morning, you can record your to-dos and go back to sleep without worrying.

- Breathe deeply and try progressive relaxation of the muscles, beginning with the feet and working your way up the body.

- When possible, let natural light wake you in the morning. If you have to wake up before dawn, use a nature or sunrise-simulating alarm clock; it will wake you gently rather than startle you.

That's right: find a way to wake up gently. One of the worst side effects of an alarm clock for some people is that it can stimulate lots of stress hormones. Waking to the sun is nature's way to get us up—gently. When our eyes detect the increased level of light at dawn, a signal is sent to the brain where the production of serotonin causes us to slowly wake up. This natural method of waking leaves us feeling refreshed and energized. Waking up to daylight or simulated daylight helps set the body's clock. The time you wake up today by light is the time your brain and body are now programmed to wake up tomorrow. Once a pattern is established with light-stimulated waking, you'll be more able to wake up at a regular time that has been set by serotonin.

At the other end of the circadian scale, darkness triggers the conversion of serotonin to melatonin. Easing your way into the darkness can be done by dimming the lights of the bedroom and bathroom and making use of candlelight! Since light governs our internal body clocks, it makes sense to use it to make us sleepy and to wake us.

GOD FIRST AND LAST

As we wake to the sunlight made by God's hands or drift off to sleep meditating on His Word, our first and last thoughts of the day should be of Him. Here's a wonderful bedtime prayer to bless you as you sleep!

> Lord Jesus, through the power of the Holy Spirit,
> go back into my memory as I sleep.
> Every hurt that has ever been done to me,
> heal that hurt.
> Every hurt that I have ever caused another person,
> heal that hurt.
> All the relationships that have been damaged in my
> whole life that I am not aware of,
> heal those relationships.
> But, Lord, if there is anything that I need to do;

if I need to go to a person because he or she is still
suffering from my hand,
bring to my awareness that person.
I choose to forgive and I ask to be forgiven.
Remove whatever bitterness may be in my heart, Lord,
and fill the empty spaces with your love.
Amen.
—Author unknown

REMEMBER!

Sleep is not optional!

- The body needs seven to nine hours of sleep (in the dark) per night for optimum health.
- The body's internal clock is regulated by lightness and darkness.
- Too much TV and other stimulants (like caffeine) before bedtime result in less sleep.
- To relax before bedtime, try herbal tea or hot milk, a hot bath, aromatherapy, and/or deep breathing.
- Keep the bedroom dark and at a comfortable temperature (approximately 70 degrees).
- Never allow a TV in the bedroom!

Remember: The body's internal clock demands a good night's sleep for health—so get it!

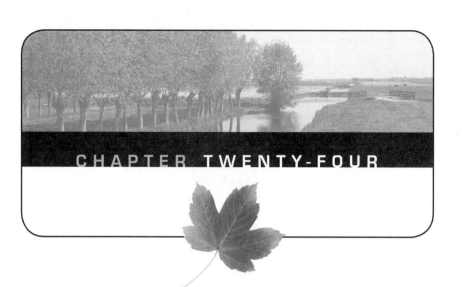

CHAPTER TWENTY-FOUR

TIME AND TIME AGAIN

●

There is a time for everything,
and a season for every activity under heaven.
—Ecclesiastes 3:1–8

IT is only with the heart that one can see rightly; what is essential is invisible to the eye." This quote is from one of my favorite books, *The Little Prince* by Antoine de Saint-Exupéry. The Little Prince learns that love is truly the most important part of life. The things and the people we love and treasure (Luke 12:34) should get the most of our time. If we really think about that and evaluate it, we may not be too happy with the way our time is currently being spent. Slowing down to smell the roses, or the spaghetti sauce, gives us more time to spend with those we love—our Creator, our spouse, our family, our friends, our neighbors. They all want time with us. Do we have time for them?

Do we have time to love ourselves? Christ in us—a precious treasure—is carried around in our jars of clay! Paul said in 2 Corinthians 4:6 that the Creator God, *"who said, 'Let light shine out of darkness,' made his light shine in our hearts"*—Christ in us. That is the way the world knows that what we do—our strength, our love—is not of ourselves, but from God.

In Creation's garden, God gave humans every provision for daily renewal of our bodies. He provided us with whole foods and rivers of water and sunshine to give us the energy and nutrients and the internal clock that our body systems and metabolism must have for health. He gave us work to do and music, dancing, and playing for physical activity that burns that energy and regulates our metabolism and chemical balance.

He gave us families and friends, whom we love and who love us. He gave us a desire to seek Him and find Him in prayer and meditation. He gave us the night, with the moon and the stars, for sleep that renews us physically, emotionally, and spiritually. God gave all this—and He gave us the time to do it. We have to take the time to know Him and His ways and trust His understanding and wisdom.

> *Trust in the LORD with all your heart*
> **and lean not on your own understanding;**
> *in all your ways acknowledge him,*
> *and he will make your paths straight.*
> **Do not be wise in your own eyes;**
> *fear the LORD and shun evil.*
> **This will bring health to your body**
> **and nourishment to your bones.**
> —Proverbs 3:5–8 (bold added)

Take time to know Him. He made you. He knows you. He loves you. He wants to give you wisdom and nourishment and health. Take time to find it.

We need to take time:

- Time to grow things to eat—if nothing else but beautiful green herbs in a window
- Time to enjoy cooking slow food and eating with family and friends
- Time for physical activity—daily work and chores or intentional exercise
- Time with God both alone and in fellowship with the body of Christ in church
- Time outdoors in the sunshine daily to enjoy the Creator's world
- Time with our spouses
- Time with our children, our families, and our friends
- Time to sleep—really sleep!

More than anything else, we must take time for the purpose for which we were created:

- Time to glorify God and enjoy Him forever
- Time to know Him through prayer and meditation and His world
- Time to spend with those He has given to us to love
- Time to take care of our bodies, which He made to be a temple, a dwelling place for His Spirit

Do you not know that your body is a temple of the Holy Spirit, who is in you, whom you have received from God? You are not your own; you were bought at a price. Therefore honor God with your body.
—1 Corinthians 6:19–20

REMEMBER!

For rest (prayer, meditation, relaxation, and sleep), choose the following:

- Prayer, meditation, and quiet time daily
- Reconnection with nature
- Quiet hobbies, like games, reading, or knitting
- Time daily with your significant other and family
- Adequate sleep

Remember: Take the time...to take time...for God, for yourself, for your family.

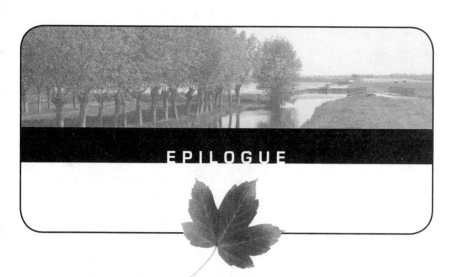

PARADISE OF GOD

He who has an ear, let him hear what the Spirit says to the churches.
*To him who overcomes, I will give the right to eat from **the tree of life,***
which is in the paradise of God.
—Revelation 2:7 (bold added)

*Then the angel showed me **the river of the water of life,***
as clear as crystal, flowing from the throne of God and of the Lamb
*down the middle of the great street of the city. **On each side of the river***
stood the tree of life, bearing twelve crops of fruit, yielding its fruit
***every month.** And the leaves of the tree are for the healing of the nations.*
***No longer will there be any curse.** The throne of God and of the Lamb*
*will be in the city, and **his servants will serve him.***
They will see his face, and his name will be on their foreheads.
There will be no more night. They will not need the light of a lamp
*or the light of the sun, for **the Lord God will give them light.***
And they will reign for ever and ever.
—Revelation 22:1–5 (bold added)

Then I heard every creature in heaven and on earth
and under the earth and on the sea, and all that is in them, singing:
"To him who sits on the throne and to the Lamb
be praise and honor and glory and power, for ever and ever!"
—Revelation 5:13 (bold added)

> *"No eye has seen,*
> *no ear has heard,*
> *no mind has conceived*
> *what God has prepared for those who love him."*
> —1 Corinthians 2:9 (bold added)

God says in Isaiah 55:8 that His thoughts are not our thoughts, nor are our ways His ways. Just as we cannot imagine the beauty that was Eden, we cannot imagine the beauty that heaven will be. The kingdom of God, the New Jerusalem, heaven—it will be a return to the paradise of God. The day that all of creation has been longing for will be here—when we are once again with God. In Isaiah 25 and 26, a word portrait of that day is painted: In that day on Mount Zion, the Lord Almighty will prepare a feast of rich food for all peoples, a banquet of the best meats and the finest wines. In that day, this song will be sung:

> *We have a strong city;*
> *God makes salvation*
> *its walls and ramparts.*
> *Open the gates*
> *that the righteous nation may enter,*
> *the nation that keeps faith.*
> *You will keep in perfect peace*
> *him whose mind is steadfast,*
> *because he trusts in you.*
> *Trust in the LORD forever, for the LORD,*
> *the LORD, is the Rock eternal.*
> —Isaiah 26:1–4

PREPARADISE—ENJOY IT NOW

> *All creatures of our God and King,*
> *Lift up your voice and with us sing.*
> —Francis of Assisi, "All Creatures of Our God and King"

Enjoy His creation now. Don't wait until tomorrow. Have your quiet time on your porch. Listen to the birds. Sing with them in praise to our Creator. Relax in the hammock. Walk in the sunshine. Play in the park with your children or grandchildren. Hold hands under the shade tree. Watch the sunset, arm in arm with your honey. Pick strawberries. Take a homebound friend to a rose garden. Grow roses or strawberries yourself. Love your neighbor; take him the roses and strawberries that you grow. Tell him about the God who made us—and all that was created for His pleasure. Tell him about the God who loved us enough to send His Son, Jesus Christ, so that man and creation would be restored to rightful fellowship with Him. All of this takes time—time for the Creator and time for His creation.

The indwelling presence of the Holy Spirit in the heart of the Christian restores God's relationship with man to that which was intended in the beginning. As His sons and His representatives on earth, we should care as He would not only for our earthly bodies, where He dwells, but also for the rest of mankind and for His world. As we seek to nourish our bodies and souls as He intended and made provision for, let us also seek to guard, care for, and tend nature. This should be a response to our knowing and understanding and loving God.

Be faithful to do His will until Christ returns and takes us to reign and worship and fellowship forever and ever with Him in **paradise**—because we were **made for paradise.**

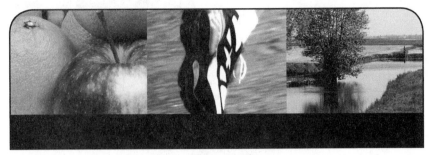

RESOURCES

HEALTHY EATING

American Dietetic Association Web site. http://www.eatright.org.

Balmuth, Deborah L. *Herb Mixtures and Spicy Blends*. Pownal, VT: Storey Publishing, 1996.

Berk, Sally Ann. *Farmer's Market Cooking*. New York: Black Dog & Leventhal Publishers, 2001.

Brown, Kathleen L., and Jeanine Pollak. *Herbal Teas: 101 Nourishing Blends for Daily Health and Vitality*. Pownal, VT: Storey Books, 1999.

Bumgarner, Marlene Anne. *The New Book of Whole Grains*. New York: St. Martin's Griffin, 1997.

Byrnes, Christine. *A Great Bowl of Soup*. New York: Sterling Publishing Company, 2006.

Cunningham, Marion; Fannie Merritt Farmer. *The Fannie Farmer Cookbook*. New York: Knopf, 1996.

Dufty, William. *Sugar Blues*. Radnor, PA: Chilton Book Company, 1975.

Ellis, Hattie. *Tea: Discovering, Exploring, Enjoying*. London; New York: Ryland Peters & Small, 2002.

Gittleman, Ann Louise. *Get the Sugar Out: 501 Simple Ways to Cut the Sugar in Any Diet*. New York: Crown Trade Paperbacks, 1996.

Greenberg, Patricia, and Helen Newton Hartung. *The Whole Soy Cookbook*. New York: Three Rivers Press, 1998.

Grimaldi, Polly. *Quick and Easy Soy and Tofu Recipes*. Hayward, CA: Bristol Publishing Enterprises, 2004.

Hill, Tony. *The Contemporary Encyclopedia of Herbs and Spices: Seasonings for the Global Kitchen*. Hoboken, NJ: John Wiley, 2004.

Johns, Pamela Sheldon. *Gelato! Italian Ice Creams, Sorbetti & Granite*. Berkeley, CA: Ten Speed Press, 2000.

Lauterbach, Barbara. *The Splendid Spoonful: From Custard to Crème Brûlée*. San Francisco: Chronicle Books, 2005.

Longacre, Doris J. *More-with-Less Cookbook*. Scottdale, PA: Herald Press, 2000.

Lund, JoAnna M., and Barbara Alpert. *Cooking Healthy with Soy*. New York: Perigee, 2005.

Madison, Deborah, and Laurie Smith. *Local Flavors*. New York: Broadway Books, 2002.

Meyerowitz, Steve. *The Organic Food Guide*. Guilford, CT: Globe Pequot, 2005.

Mozian, Laurie Deutsch. *Foods That Fight Disease*. New York: Avery, 2000.

Perry, Sara. *The New Tea Book: A Guide to Black, Green, Herbal, and Chai Tea*. San Francisco: Chronicle Books, 2001.

Petusevsky, Steve. *The Whole Foods Market Cookbook*. New York: Clarkson Potter, 2002.

Planck, Nina. *Real Food: What to Eat and Why*. New York: Bloomsbury Publisher, 2006.

Pratt, Steven, and Kathy Matthews. *Superfoods Rx*. New York: William Morrow, 2004.

Puente, Debbie. *Elegantly Easy Crème Brûlée & Other Custard Desserts*. Los Angeles: Renaissance Books, 1998.

Steward, H. Leighton. *The New Sugar Busters! Cut Sugar to Trim Fat*. New York: Ballantine Books, 2003.

Traunfeld, Jerry. *The Herbal Kitchen: Cooking with Fragrance and Flavor*. New York: William Morrow, 2005.

United States Department of Agriculture (USDA). Food Guide Pyramid. http://www.mypyramid.gov.

United States Department of Health and Human Services (HHS) and Department of Agriculture (USDA). *Dietary Guidelines for Americans 2005*. http://www.healthierus.gov/dietaryguidelines.

Vinton, Sherri Brooks, and Ann Clark Espuelas. *The Real Food Revival: Aisle by Aisle, Morsel by Morsel*. New York: Jeremy P. Tarcher/Penguin, 2005.

Wallstin, Donna, and Katherine Dieter. *Granola Madness: The Ultimate Granola Cookbook*. Novato, CA: New World Library, 1996.

Zak, Victoria. *20,000 Secrets of Tea: The Most Effective Ways to Benefit from Nature's Healing Herbs*. New York: Bantam, 2000.

PHYSICAL ACTIVITY

Anderson, Bob. *Stretching in the Office*. Bolinas, CA: Shelter Publications, 2002.

Baechle, Thomas R., Roger W. Earle, and the National Strength and Conditioning Association. *Essentials of Strength Training and Conditioning*. Champaign, IL: Human Kinetics, 2000.

Barnett, Larkin. *Functional Fitness: The Ultimate Fitness Program for Life on the Run*. Gainesville, FL: Florida Academic Press, 2006.

Brill, Patricia A. *Functional Fitness for Older Adults*. Champaign, IL: Human Kinetics, 2004.

Lyons, Pat, and Debby Burgard. *Great Shape: The First Fitness Guide for Large Women*. Lincoln, NE: IUniverse.com, 2000, 1990.

Siler, Brooke. *The Pilates Body: The Ultimate at Home Guide to Strengthening, Lengthening, and Toning Your Body—Without Machines*. New York: Broadway Books, 2000.

Westcott, Wayne L. *Strength Training for Seniors*. Champaign, IL: Human Kinetics, 1999.

Zeer, Darrin. *Office Yoga: 75 Simple Stretches for Busy People*. San Francisco, CA: Chronicle Books, 2005.

REST

Chapman, Gary. *The Five Love Languages*. Chicago: Northfield, 1995.

Cousins, Norman. *Anatomy of an Illness as Perceived by the Patient*. New York: Norton, 1979.

Dale, Melissa, Emmanuelle Lipsky, and Kellie Canning. *Aromatherapy in the Kitchen: Fragrant Foods for Body, Mind and Spirit*. Pleasant Grove, UT: Woodland Publishing, 2002.

Goings, Nanette. *Stirring Up a World of Fun*. Birmingham, AL: New Hope Publishers, 2006.

Jacke, Dave, and Eric Toensmeier. *Edible Forest Gardens*. White River Junction, VT: Chelsea Green Publishing Company, 2005.

Katz, Lawrence C., and Manning Rubin. *Keep Your Brain Alive: 83 Neurobic Exercises to Help Prevent Memory Loss and Increase Mental Fitness*. New York: Workman Publishing, 1999.

Logue, Victoria, and Frank Logue. *The Appalachian Trail Backpacker*. Birmingham, AL: Menasha Ridge Press, 2001.

Louv, Richard. *Last Child in the Woods*. Chapel Hill, NC: Algonquin Books of Chapel Hill, 2006.

Marzollo, Jean, and Walter Wick. "I Spy" collection. New York: Scholastic Readers.

De Saint-Exupéry, Antoine. *The Little Prince*. San Diego: Harcourt, 2000.

Thomas, Dian. *Recipes for Roughing It Easy*. Cincinnati, OH: Betterway, 2001.

Weinstein, Miriam. *The Surprising Power of Family Meals: How Eating Together Makes Us Smarter, Stronger, Healthier, and Happier*. Hanover, NH: Steerforth Press, 2005.

New Hope® Publishers is a division of WMU®,
an international organization
that challenges Christian believers to understand
and be radically involved in God's mission.
For more information about WMU, go to www.wmu.com.
More information about New Hope books
may be found at www.newhopepublishers.com.
New Hope books may be purchased at your local bookstore.

YOU MAY Enjoy

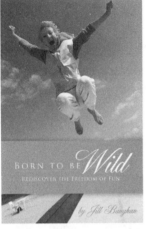

Born to Be Wild
Rediscover the Freedom of Fun
Jill Baughan
ISBN 1-59669-048-8

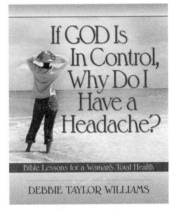

**If God Is In Control,
Why Do I Have a Headache?**
Bible Lessons for a Woman's Total Health
Debbie Taylor Williams
ISBN 1-56309-819-9

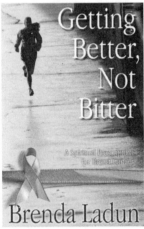

Getting Better, Not Bitter
*A Spiritual Prescription
for Breast Cancer*
Brenda Ladun
ISBN 1-56309-733-8

Available in bookstores everywhere

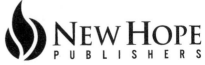

NEW HOPE
P U B L I S H E R S

For information about these books or any New Hope product, visit **www.newhopepublishers.com**.